Occupational Therapy
Pocket Guide

LYNDSEY E. JARVIS, MSOT, OTR/L

ELSEVIER

Elsevier
3251 Riverport Lane
St. Louis, Missouri 63043

OCCUPATIONAL THERAPY POCKET GUIDE   ISBN: 978-0-323-93500-5

Senior Content Strategist: Lauren Willis
Senior Content Development Specialist: Rishabh Gupta
Publishing Services Manager: Deepthi Unni
Project Manager: Sheik Mohideen K
Senior Book Designer: Renee Duenow

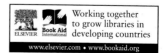

Working together
to grow libraries in
developing countries

www.elsevier.com • www.bookaid.org

Printed in India
Last digit is the print number: 9   8   7   6   5   4   3   2   1

CONTENTS

OT EVALUATION QUICK REFERENCE

VITALS
- Blood pressure
- Pulse
- Temperature
- Oxygen
- Respiration rate

ADLs
- Feeding
- Eating/swallowing
- Dressing
- Bathing
- Toileting/continence
- Hygiene/grooming
- Sexual activity

IADLs
- Cleaning
- Meal preparation
- Laundry
- Shopping
- Medication management
- Health management
- Financial management
- Driving/community mobility
- Sleep/rest
- Social participation
- Care of others
- Leisure
- Communication

FUNCTIONAL MOBILITY
- MR-ADL
- Community mobility
- Transfers
  - Chair/wheelchair
  - Couch/recliner
  - Shower/tub
  - Bed
  - Car

BALANCE
- Static sitting
- Dynamic sitting
- Static standing
- Dynamic standing

STRENGTH
- Manual muscle test

RANGE OF MOTION
- Goniometry
- Functional range of motion
  - Feed self
  - Brush hair
  - Pull up pants
  - Don shoes
  - Personal hygiene
  - Reach into cupboards/closet

COORDINATION
- Fine motor
- Gross motor

SENSORY
- Light touch
- Pain
- Proprioception
- Temperature

PERCEPTUAL/COGNITIVE
- Visual fields
- Visuo-spatial
- Visual acuity
- Visual attention and scanning
- Orientation
- Memory
- Attention span
- Problem solving
- Motor planning

ADAPTIVE EQUIPMENT/ DURABLE MEDICAL EQUIPMENT
- Individual basis

QUESTIONS
- Orientation
- Prior level of function
- Home setting
- Hobbies/interests
- Goals for therapy

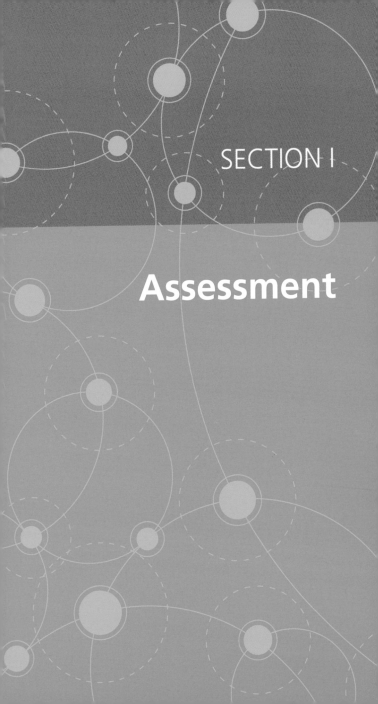

SECTION I

Assessment

Vitals

NORMAL RANGE	
BLOOD PRESSURE	<120/<80 mm Hg
PULSE	60–100 BPM
TEMPERATURE	97–99.1°F
RESPIRATORY RATE	12–20 breaths/min
OXYGEN SATURATION (SPO$_2$)	95–100%

BP	SYSTOLIC/DIASTOLIC	IMPLICATIONS*
NORMAL	<120/< 80 mm Hg	Safe for activity
HYPOTENSIVE	<90/<60 mm Hg	Not safe for activity
ELEVATED	120–129/80–89 mm Hg	Safe for activity
HYPERTENSION (HTN) STAGE 1	130–139/80–89 mm Hg	Safe for activity
HTN STAGE 2	140–160/90–100 mm Hg	Avoid vigorous activity
VERY HIGH	160–200/100–120 mm Hg	No activity, potentially enact emergency medical services (EMS)
EMERGENCY	>200/>120 mm Hg	Enact EMS

PULSE	
NORMAL	60–100 BPM
BRADYCARDIA	<60 BPM
TACHYCARDIA	>100 BPM

OXYGEN	
NORMAL	≥95%
CHRONIC OBSTRUCTIVE PULMONARY DISEASE (COPD) TARGET RANGE	88–92%
HYPOXIC	85–95%
SEVERELY HYPOXIC	<85%

*Intended to provide general guidance; always use specific parameters as set forth by the referring MD.

Range of Motion

SHOULDER	
Flexion	0°–170°/180°
Extension	0°–60°
Abduction	0°–170°/180°
Horizontal Abduction	0°–40°
Horizontal Adduction	0°–130°
Internal Rotation	0°–70°
External Rotation	0°–90°

ELBOW	
Flexion	0°–135°/150°
Supination	0°–80°/90°
Pronation	0°–80°/90°

WRIST	
Flexion	0°–80°
Extension	0°–70°
Ulnar Deviation	0°–30°
Radial Deviation	0°–20°

FINGERS	
MCP Flexion	0°–90°
MCP Hyperextension	0°–15°/45°
PIP Flexion	0°–110°
DIP Flexion	0°–80°
Abduction	0°–25°

DIP, Distal interphalangeal; *MCP,* metacarpophalangeal; *PIP,* proximal interphalangeal.

THUMB	
MCP Flexion	0°–50°
IP Flexion	0°–80°/90°
Abduction	0°–50°

IP, Interphalangeal; *MCP*, metacarpophalangeal.

HIP	
Flexion	0°–120°
Extension	0°–30°
Abduction	0°–40°
Adduction	0°–35°
Internal Rotation	0°–45°
External Rotation	0°–45°

KNEE	
Flexion	0°–135°

ANKLE/FOOT	
Plantar Flexion	0°–50°
Dorsiflexion	0°–15°
Inversion	0°–35°
Eversion	0°–20°

Muscle Grades

MUSCLE GRADES		
0	Zero	No muscle contraction detected
1	Trace	Contraction is felt or visible but no movement occurs
2−	Poor−	Movement through partial range of motion (ROM) in gravity-eliminated plane
2	Poor	Movement through full ROM in gravity-eliminated plane
2+	Poor+	Movement through <50% ROM against gravity
3−	Fair−	Movement through >50% ROM against gravity
3	Fair	Movement through full ROM against gravity
3+	Fair+	Movement through full ROM with slight pressure
4−	Good−	Movement through full ROM and holds test position against slight to moderate pressure
4	Good	Movement through full ROM and holds test position against moderate to strong pressure
5	Normal	Holds test position against strong pressure

Adapted from Palmer and Epler (1998).

4

Balance Grades

STATIC SITTING BALANCE	
Poor−	Requires maximal assistance to maintain sitting balance
Poor	Requires moderate assistance to maintain sitting balance
Poor+	Requires minimal assistance to maintain sitting balance
Fair−	Maintains sitting balance with upper extremity (UE) support only
Fair	Maintains sitting balance unsupported, without assistance or UE support
Fair+	Maintains sitting balance against minimal pressure with limited postural sway
Good−	Maintains sitting balance against moderate pressure with limited postural sway
Good	Maintains sitting balance against maximal pressure with limited postural sway
Normal	Maintains sitting balance against maximal pressure with no postural sway
DYNAMIC SITTING BALANCE	
Poor−	Requires maximal assistance to right self, ipsilateral reach to front only
Poor	Requires moderate assistance to right self, ipsilateral reach to front only
Poor+	Requires minimal assistance to right self, ipsilateral reach to front and side
Fair−	Able to right self with UE support only, ipsilateral reach to front and side
Fair	Able to right self independently, performs minimal weight shifts

Fair+	Able to right self independently, performs minimal weight shifts, crosses midline minimally
Good−	Able to right self independently, performs moderate weight shifts, crosses midline moderately, engages in seated activity
Good	Able to right self independently, performs moderate weight shifts, crosses midline maximally, reaches in all directions
Normal	Able to right self independently, performs maximal weight shifts, reaches/leans outside base of support, independent with all seated activity

STATIC STANDING BALANCE	
Poor−	Requires maximal assistance and UE support to maintain standing balance
Poor	Requires moderate assistance and UE support to maintain standing balance
Poor+	Requires minimal assistance and UE support to maintain standing balance
Fair−	Requires UE support and contact guard assist (CGA) to maintain standing balance
Fair	Maintains standing balance for 1–2 min without UE support. Requires UE support for longer-standing duration
Fair+	Maintains standing balance against minimal pressure with limited postural sway
Good−	Maintains standing balance against moderate pressure with limited postural sway
Good	Maintains standing balance against maximal pressure with limited postural sway
Normal	Maintains standing balance against maximal pressure with no postural sway

DYNAMIC STANDING BALANCE	
Poor−	Requires maximal assistance and UE support to maintain position
Poor	Requires moderate assistance and UE support to maintain position, reaches ipsilaterally
Poor+	Requires minimal assistance and UE support to maintain position, reaches ipsilaterally

ASSESSMENT

Fair−	Requires CGA and UE support to maintain position, reaches ipsilaterally, performs minimal weight shifts
Fair	Does not require assistance but must use UE support to maintain position, reaches ipsilaterally, performs minimal weight shifts
Fair+	Requires UE support to maintain position, maintains balance while turning head/trunk, crosses midline minimally, performs moderate weight shifts
Good−	Maintains position independently, without support, crosses midline moderately, performs moderate weight shifts, accepts minimal pressure
Good	Maintains position independently, without support, crosses midline maximally, accepts moderate pressure, maintains balance while picking up an object from floor
Normal	Maintains position independently, without support, crosses midline maximally, accepts maximal pressure, can shift weight easily in all directions

5

Orthostatic Hypotension

ORTHOSTATC HYPOTENSION

1. Patient should rest for a few minutes before blood pressure (BP) and pulse are measured

2. First, measure BP and pulse in a supine position

3. Next, have the patient sit on the edge of the bed and take both BP and pulse in a sitting position within 1–2 min

4. Then, have patient stand and take both BP and pulse in a standing position within 1–2 min

5. Note any symptoms with transfer

6. A decrease in systolic of $\geq$20 mm Hg, or in diastolic of $\geq$10 mm Hg, and/or an increase in pulse of $\geq$20 BPM from supine to standing is considered abnormal and should be reported to MD

7. If orthostatic hypotension (OH) is confirmed, further readings can be taken at 5 min, 10 min, etc. to provide further information regarding rate of recovery

6

Pitting Edema

GRADE	DEPTH	LENGTH OF TIME SKIN STAYS PITTED
1+	2 mm	Resolves almost immediately
2+	4 mm	About 5 s
3+	6 mm	About 10–15 s
4+	8 mm	>20 s

Initial Interview

7

ASSESSMENT

PRIOR TO EVALUATION

- Confirm that a current and signed order for occupational therapy (OT) evaluation and treatment is in the patient's chart.
- Review the patient's chart for medical history, reason for OT referral, precautions, contraindications, labs, and medications relevant to current medical status.
- Gather necessary supplies (e.g., gait belt, walker, blood pressure cuff, pulse oximeter, goniometer, gloves, and personal protective equipment [PPE]).
- Obtain assistance from additional staff if necessary for patient and employee safety.
- Perform hand hygiene and observe applicable universal precautions.

INITIAL INTERVIEW

ORIENTATION

- What is your name? (Person)
- Where are you? (Place)
- What is the date/time of day? (Time)
- Do you know why you are in the hospital/skilled nursing facility (SNF)? (Situation)
  - Documented as (example): Patient is alert and oriented to person and place, or patient is A&O x2

PRIOR LEVEL OF FUNCTION

- Assistance for activities of daily living (ADLs)/instrumental activities of daily living (IADLs)
  - How much assistance was required to complete self-care activities?

13

- How much assistance was required for household chores such as cleaning, laundry, meal preparation, and medication management?
- Who provided the assistance (e.g., family, paid caregiver, neighbor)?
- If employing paid caregiving services, how many hours per day/week?
- Did you use any adaptive equipment?
- What type of ambulation device was used indoors and outdoors?
- Community mobility
  - Were you still driving?
  - Did you require a chaperone for outings?

HOME ENVIRONMENT

- Do you live in a house, apartment, assisted living facility, or adult family home?
- How many steps to enter?
- How many floor levels are in the home? On which floor are bedrooms and bathrooms located?
- Are there any barriers, architecturally or otherwise, that cause difficulty with daily activities?
- Do you have any existing adaptive equipment/durable medical equipment?
- Are there any other people living in the home?
- Are there any pets in the home?

GETTING TO KNOW THE PATIENT

- What is your daily routine?
- What are your roles (e.g., family, vocational)?
- Do you have a support system (e.g., family, friends, neighbors, community)?
- What are your hobbies and interests?
- Are there any occupations or preferences related to your culture, religion, or spirituality that you would like to discuss?

GOALS FOR THERAPY/CLIENT-CENTERED CARE

- What activities would you like to improve upon with therapy, and how would you prioritize those activities from most to least important?

- If a patient has difficulty answering this question, s/he can be prompted by asking what occupations s/he needs to do, wants to do, and is expected to do.
- Are there any other areas you feel I have missed that you would like to discuss?

8

Analysis of Occupational Performance

ANALYSIS OF OCCUPATIONAL PERFORMANCE

A comprehensive performance analysis focuses on the dynamic relationship between the patient, environment, and occupation, and is thus highly individualized. Additionally, a great deal of variation exists between the different ways in which patients carry out activities of daily living (ADLs) based on personal preference and numerous other client factors. The following examples demonstrate the performance of one such possibility, and are meant to serve as a **basic** analysis only, with a focus on motor skills and movement-related functions. Skilled clinical judgment should be used to identify ineffective motor planning and performance skills in order to guide specific intervention.

Phrasing can be modified and adapted for use in documentation.

FEEDING AND DEGLUTITION

For full dysphagia assessment see Conditions: Dysphagia

- Identify adaptive equipment needs:
  - Built-up handles
  - Lightweight or weighted utensils
  - Curved/offset utensils
  - Rocker knife
  - Scoop plate
  - Plate guard
  - Swivel spoon
  - Nosey cup
  - Plates/bowls with suction pad
  - Universal-cuff (U-cuff)

- Liftware
- Readi-Steadi Anti-Tremor Glove
- Proper positioning:
  - In chair:
    - Patient sits with hips flexed 75°–100° to prevent sacral sitting (this can cause a kyphotic thoracic cavity and consequently interfere with the ability to swallow).
    - Knees flexed to 90° with feet resting on flat surface.
  - In bed:
    - Hips flexed to 90° (a wedge under knees can assist with this position).
  - Adequate sitting balance to maintain midline, or use of lateral supports to maintain position.
- Pre-oral phase:
  - Cuts food on plate: Knife and fork are held with a pronated grasp. The index finger is extended, placing pressure along the top of each utensil. The nondominant hand steadies the fork while the dominant hand moves back and forth creating a cutting motion that is generated through shoulder flexion and extension in internal rotation.
  - Loads fork and spoon: Lateral pincer grasp with wrist supinated to hold spoon or fork for scooping, or pronated grasp to stab food with fork.
  - Produces smooth transit to mouth: The forearm moves in a pronation to supination pattern when bringing food to mouth. Movement is smooth to prevent spillage from utensil. Orients mouth (timing and opening of jaw) to receive food.
- Oral phase: (Voluntary)
  - Adequate secretion management to produce bolus formation and to prevent pocketing.
  - Adequate sensation to avoid biting cheeks or tongue and to discern proper temperature.
  - Effective oral-motor function to facilitate coordinated movement of jaw (mastication), tongue, lips, and cheeks for formation of an optimal size bolus.
  - Tongue elevation to compress the bolus against the hard palate, while the posterior part of the tongue creates a chute allowing the bolus to pass into the oropharynx.

ASSESSMENT

- Pharyngeal phase: (Involuntary)
  - Soft palate elevates to close off the nasopharynx.
  - Epiglottis covers the larynx, which contracts along with the vocal folds to temporarily halt respiration in order to protect the airway by preventing food from entering the trachea.
  - Upper esophageal sphincter opens.
- Esophageal phase: (Involuntary)
  - Bolus is moved into the stomach through rhythmic contractions of the esophagus (peristalsis). The upper esophageal sphincter prevents food from reentering into the mouth and the lower esophageal sphincter causes food to remain in the stomach preventing regurgitation.
- Ability to sit upright for 1 hour after eating:
  - Sits at an upright angle of at least 60° to prevent silent aspiration from reflux. This is especially important for patients at higher risk of aspirating or with gastroesophageal reflux disease (GERD).

TOILETING

- Identify adaptive equipment needs:
  - Bidet
  - Handheld bidet sprayer
  - Long-handled wiping aid
    - **Toilet transfer:** Riser, bedside commode, safety frame, electronic toilet lift, grab bars, stand-alone toilet safety rail, flip-up grab bar, transfer pole, slide board, sit to stand lift, transfer pivot disc.
- Maintains standing balance, or if seated, produces sufficient weight shift side to side in order to manage clothing over hips:
  - Integration of adequate visual, vestibular, and somatosensory (proprioception/exteroception) processing systems.
  - Effective postural strategies: Produces corrective/stabilizing response.
  - Adequate muscle strength.
  - Alternates grasp on bilateral upper extremity support or releases grasp bilaterally in order to pull pants and undergarments down.
  - Elbow flexion with shoulder extension and fine motor (FM) coordination to grasp pants. Elbow extension and trunk flexion to lower pants.

- Volitional pelvic floor contraction and relaxation for bowel and bladder elimination.
- Perineal cleaning post bowel movement:
  - FM coordination for folding paper.
  - Sufficient knee and trunk flexion to weight shift forward.
  - Shoulder internal rotation with extension and adduction to reach perineal area.
  - Adequate grasp of toilet paper with radial and ulnar wrist deviation for wiping.
  - Visual acuity for inspection of toilet paper to ensure thoroughness.
- Sit to stand with ability to bring pants and undergarments up over hips:
  - Trunk flexion with knee extension to weight shift forward and lift into partial standing.
  - FM coordination to grasp pants and undergarments, pulling them up over hips, prior to trunk extension.

BATHING

- Identify durable medical equipment/adaptive equipment needs:
  - Shower chair
  - Anchored grab bars
  - Handheld shower head
  - Suction-cup handheld shower head holder
  - Nonskid mat inside shower
  - Rubber-backed mat outside of shower
  - Silicone hair scrubber
  - No-rinse shampoo cap
  - Foot scrubbing pad
  - Long-handled sponge
  - Long-handled lotion applicator
  - Hair funnel for upright bathing
  - **Shower or tub transfer:** Tub transfer bench, bath lift, sliding transfer bench, anchored grab bars, transfer pole, rolling shower chair. If patient has sliding glass doors with tub, these can typically be replaced with rod and curtain. If feasible, recommend replacing bathtub with walk-in shower.

- Item retrieval and transport:
  - Opens and reaches into drawers or closet, accesses items at various heights, carries towel and clothing, or transports with ambulation device.
- **Dons/doffs clothing:** (Addressed in subsequent section)
- **Shower transfer:** (Will vary depending on shower configuration and use of durable medical equipment)
- Operates water volume lever and temperature control:
  - Adequate shoulder flexion, forearm supination/pronation, and power grasp to turn levers. Intact sensation to discern appropriate water temperature.
- Maintains standing or seated balance:
  - Integration of adequate visual, vestibular, and somatosensory (proprioception/exteroception) processing systems.
  - Effective postural strategies: Produces corrective/stabilizing response throughout activity.
- Washes hair and body:
  - Adequate grasp and FM coordination to open bottles, hold soap, and washcloth.
  - Sufficient range of motion (ROM) including shoulder and elbow flexion with proximal interphalangeal (PIP)/distal interphalangeal (DIP) isolation to rub shampoo around scalp/hair and rinse.
- Washes perineal area:
  - Stands with wide base of support (BOS).
  - Elbow and wrist flexion with pronation and FM coordination to thoroughly clean perineal area.
  - Shoulder extension with adduction and wrist flexion to reach behind.
  - Attention to direction of wiping to prevent bacteria (due to excrement, if present) from entering the urethra, especially for female patients.
- Rinse and dry:
  - Sufficient strength/ROM to move handheld showerhead over head and body or ability to turn self under mounted shower head. Grasps and wraps towel around body.

DRESSING

- Identify adaptive equipment needs:
  - Dressing stick
  - Long- or short-handled reacher

- Sock aid
- Compression stocking donner
- Long-handled shoehorn
- Foot funnel
- Button hook
- Magnetic button adaptors
- Zipper pull rings
- No tie/elastic laces
- Velcro clothing
- Clip and pull dressing aid
- A transfer pole can be utilized when standing to pull clothes up over hips
- Clothing retrieval and transport:
  - Opens drawers or closet, reaches for clothing at various heights, carries or transports with use of walker.
- Dons shirt:
  - Identifies front and back of clothing.
  - FM coordination to bunch material.
  - Shoulder flexion with elbow flexion/extension to thread arms through opening of sleeves.
  - Trunk, shoulder, elbow, neck flexion with grasp of shirt to pull overhead.
  - Shoulder internal rotation, elbow/wrist flexion and grasp to bring shirt down over trunk.
- Dons pants/undergarments:
  - Grasps top of pants.
  - Hip, knee, ankle flexion to raise foot.
  - Shoulder flexion, elbow extension to bring pants to foot.
  - Knee/hip extension to thread leg into pants.
  - Repeat for second leg with hip external rotation prior to threading leg through pants.
  - Trunk flexion with knee extension to lift into partial standing.
  - Grasps pants and undergarments, pulling up over hips simultaneously with trunk extension.
- Dons socks/shoes:
  - Trunk, hip, knee, ankle flexion to raise foot. Shoulder flexion, elbow extension to bring sock/shoe to foot.
  - Lateral grasp of sock or shoe to pull onto foot.
  - FM coordination to tie laces.

HYGIENE AND GROOMING

- Identify adaptive equipment needs:
  - Electronic toothbrush
  - Floss aid
  - Lightweight or weighted hairbrush
  - Long-handled hairbrush
  - Long-handled lotion applicator
  - Long-handled swivel head nail clippers
  - Suction brush (for hands and under nails)
  - Suction denture brush
  - Universal-cuff (U-cuff) for holding implements
  - Long-handled razor
  - Self-inspection mirror
- Washes hands:
  - Shoulder and elbow flexion with forearm pronation to reach forward. Grasps and turns faucet handle for appropriate water temperature and pressure.
  - Coordinates bilateral upper extremity (BUE) movement to express soap onto hand.
  - Shoulder internal rotation, elbow flexion, wrist/MCP/PIP/DIP flexion and extension to rub hands together for lather of soap and to rinse under water.
- Brushes and flosses teeth:
  - Neat pincer grasp to maintain hold of floss. Shoulder flexion, abduction, internal rotation with elbow flexion to bring hands to mouth. DIP isolation to manipulate floss between teeth.
  - Shoulder flexion, abduction, internal rotation, elbow/wrist flexion with ulnar deviation to place toothbrush in mouth. Grasps toothbrush with rotational wrist movement and coordinated horizontal abduction/adduction movement of shoulder to move brush over teeth.
  - Trunk flexion to bring head over sink, cups hand or grasps cup, bringing to mouth in order to rinse.
  - Closure of mouth with coordinated oral buccal lingual movements to swish water around mouth and spit into sink.
- Shaves:
  - Shoulder and elbow flexion with forearm pronation to reach forward. Grasps and turns faucet handle for appropriate water temperature and pressure. Forearm

supination to place palms under water. Elbow flexion to reach toward face with FM control to dampen skin. Bilateral FM coordination to manipulate shaving cream container. Wrist, MCP, PIP, DIP extension with FM control to lather shaving cream and rub on face.

- Shoulder flexion, abduction, internal rotation, elbow flexion with wrist flexion/extension movements to shave face with appropriate grasp and pressure of razor. Bilateral coordination to keep skin taut. Trunk flexion to lean over sink throughout activity. Visual acuity to ensure thoroughness.
- Brushes/combs hair:
  - Grasps brush or comb. Shoulder flexion/external rotation with elbow flexion and wrist radial and ulnar deviation with horizontal abduction to produce brushing motion. Shoulder flexion, adduction with elbow/wrist flexion and supination to reach opposite side of head.

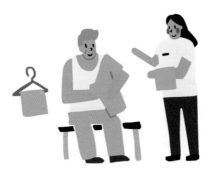

9

Common Upper Extremity Conditions With Special Orthopedic Tests

ROTATOR CUFF TEAR

Sign or symptom: Pain in side of shoulder and difficulty performing flexion, abduction, and external rotation.

Test: Drop Arm Test

Procedure: Occupational therapist (OT) passively abducts shoulder to 90° with palm facing down. From this position, patient is instructed to lower arm slowly and in a controlled manner.

Positive findings: Inability to lower arm with good motor control.

Additional tests: Lateral Jobe Test, strength of <3/5 for shoulder abduction or external rotation.

ROTATOR CUFF TENDINITIS

Sign or symptom: Pain in anterior and lateral aspect of shoulder/arm that typically does not extend below elbow, painful movement in scapular plane.

Test: Exam of shoulder

Procedure: Palpate tendons of supraspinatus and infraspinatus. Perform manual muscle testing of scapular plane abduction and external rotation.

Positive findings: Pain when palpating tendons and with muscle testing. Nonpainful passive range of motion.

Additional tests: Check history for occupations that may cause repetitive strain or stress.

ADHESIVE CAPSULITIS

Sign or symptom: Progressive reduction in range of motion, pain often reported near insertion of deltoid.

Test: Exam of shoulder

Procedure: Assess for loss of both active and passive range of motion.

Positive findings: Capsular pattern of external rotation being most limited, followed by abduction and, to a lesser degree, flexion and internal rotation.

Additional tests: Shoulder Shrug Sign, check history for any prolonged period of shoulder immobilization.

THORACIC OUTLET SYNDROME

Sign or symptom: Pain in neck/upper extremity, numbness or tingling with worsening symptoms during activity above shoulder level.

Test: Adson's Test

Procedure: Patient turns head toward affected side and slightly extends neck. OT passively abducts shoulder to 30° and externally rotates, then, while monitoring pulse, brings shoulder into extension.

Positive findings: Diminished radial pulse.

Additional tests: Roos Test

SUBACHROMIAL IMPINGEMENT SYNDROME

Sign or symptom: Pain in neck and arm, weakness, difficulty reaching behind back and with overhead activity.

Test: Neer's Test

Procedure: OT stabilizes scapula and passively flexes and internally rotates shoulder. Test variation includes neutral position rather than internally rotated.

Positive findings: Painful arc between 60° and 120° of flexion.

Additional tests: Hawkin's Test, Jobe's Test/Empty Can Test, Painful Arc Test.

CUBITAL TUNNEL SYNDROME

Sign or symptom: Paresthesia, weakness, and pain along path of ulnar nerve below elbow and in ulnar nerve distribution of hand.

Test: Ulnar Nerve Compression Test

Procedure: With elbow flexed 20°, OT palpates the ulnar nerve just lateral to the medial epicondyle. Pressure is held for 60 s.

Positive findings: Pain and/or paresthesia in ulnar nerve distribution.

Additional tests: Tinel's Sign at elbow, Elbow Flexion Test.

LATERAL EPICONDYLITIS/TENNIS ELBOW

Sign or symptom: Lateral elbow pain that radiates down forearm and wrist, decreased grip strength.

Test: Cozen's Test

Procedure: With arm supported and elbow slightly flexed, instruct patient to pronate forearm, extend and radially deviate wrist. OT places pressure over lateral epicondyle and, with other hand, provides resistance against wrist extension.

Positive findings: Pain in lateral epicondyle.

Additional tests: Mill's Test, Maudsley's Test.

CARPAL TUNNEL SYNDROME

Sign or symptom: Paresthesia, weakness, and pain in median nerve distribution, typically described as burning or electrical shock sensation.

Test: Tinel's Sign at wrist

Procedure: OT taps over transverse carpal ligament.

Positive findings: Paresthesia in median nerve distribution.

Additional tests: Phalen's Test, Reverse Phalen's Test, Carpal Compression Test.

ULNAR NERVE PALSY

Sign or symptom: Loss of sensation in ulnar nerve distribution, weakness, loss of coordination and grip strength.

Test: Froment's Sign (assesses strength of adductor pollicis)

Procedure: Patient holds piece of paper between thumb and index finger by adducting thumb against index finger. OT attempts to pull paper from grip.

Positive findings: Paper slips out or patient attempts to compensate by flexing interphalangeal (IP) joint of thumb.

Additional tests: Jeanne's Sign, Wartenberg's Sign.

Mobility and Balance Assessments

PURPOSE	FEATURES	TIME	INTERPRETATION OF SCORES
SIX-MINUTE WALK TEST (6 MWT) (Free[a])			
Cardiovascular test that measures functional status, exercise capacity, response to surgical intervention, and progress with therapy.	Patient walks as far as possible in 6 min.	<10 min	Age norms: (In meters) • 60–69 y/o M = 572 F = 538 • 70–79 y/o M = 527 F =471 • 80–89 y/o M = 417 F = 392

Adapted From Academy of Neurologic Physical Therapy. (n.d.). *Six-Minute Walk Test (6MWT)*. Retrieved April 30, 2023, from https://www.neuropt.org/docs/default-source/cpgs/core-outcome-measures/6mwt-pocket-guide-proof9.pdf?sfvrsn59ee25043_0

FIVE TIMES SIT-TO-STAND (Free[a])			
Assesses fall risk, lower extremity strength, and transitional movement strategies.	Patient completes five sit-to-stand intervals as quickly as possible.	<5 min	Age norms: (In seconds) • 60–69 y/o 11.4 • 70–79 y/o 12.6 • 80–89 y/o 14.8

Data from Five Times Sit to Stand Test. (n.d.). *AbilityLab*. https://www.sralab.org/rehabilitation-measures/five-times-sit-stand-test

TIMED UP AND GO TEST (TUG) (Free[a])			
Provides a basic estimate of mobility status, fall risk, and balance.	Patient stands from chair, walks 10 feet at a comfortable pace, turns and walks back to chair, returning to a seated position.	<5 min	Age norms: (In seconds) • 60–69 y/o 8.1 • 70–79 y/o 9.2 • 80–89 y/o 11.3

Data from Bohannon, R. W. (2006). Reference values for the timed up and go test: a descriptive meta-analysis. *PubMed*. https://pubmed.ncbi.nlm.nih.gov/16914068/

PURPOSE	FEATURES	TIME	INTERPRETATION OF SCORES
MODIFIED CLINICAL TEST OF SENSORY INTERACTION ON BALANCE (CTSIB-M) (Free[a])			
Balance test that identifies the effectiveness of three sensory inputs including visual, vestibular, and somatosensory.	Patient is tested under four conditions to challenge different balance systems including 1. Eyes open firm surface 2. Eyes closed firm surface 3. Eyes open foam surface 4. Eyes closed foam surface	10 min	If patient performs poorly in condition 1: Visual, vestibular, and somatosensory may be compromised. 2: Vestibular and/or somatosensory may be compromised. 3: Visual and/or vestibular may be compromised. 4: Vestibular system may be compromised

Data from Reliability and validity of the mCTSIB dynamic platform test to assess balance in a population of older women living in the community. (2020). *PubMed Central (PMC)*. https://www.ncbi.nlm.nih.gov/pmc/articles/PMC728 8384/

BERG BALANCE SCALE (BBS) (Free[a])

Gold-standard test of seated/standing balance including both static and dynamic tasks.	Patient is tested on 14 tasks, rated 0–4 points for performance per task that range from sit to stand transfer to turning 360°	15–20 min	• >50 = No AD • 45–49 = Cane • 41–44 = FWW • 20–40 = FWW + assist • <45 = At risk for falls

Data from Berg Balance Scale. (2020, June 30). *Shirley Ryan AbilityLab*. https://www.sralab.org/rehabilitation-measures/berg-balance-scale

TINETTI BALANCE AND GAIT ASSESSMENT, ALSO KNOWN AS PERFORMANCE-ORIENTED MOBILITY ASSESSMENT (Free[a])

Assesses static and dynamic balance as well as gait quality. Excellent predictive validity regarding fall risk.	Divided into two sections 1. Balance: Consisting of nine components 2. Gait: Analyzes quality of gait pattern	15 min	Fall risk: • 25–28 = Low • 19–24 = Mod • <19 = High

AD, ambulation device; *FWW*, front wheeled walker.
Data from Tinetti Test. (n.d.). *Physiopedia*. Retrieved September 5, 2021, from https://www.physio-pedia.com/Tinetti_Test

ASSESSMENT

FUNCTIONAL REACH TEST (Free[a])			
A simple assessment of fall risk and balance measured by limits of stability.	Performance-based task whereby patient flexes upper extremity to 90° and reaches as far forward as possible without losing balance.	2 min	<ul><li><6" indicates a significant risk for falls.</li><li>6–10" indicates a moderate risk for falls.</li><li>Age-related norms:</li><li>41–69</li><li>Men: 14.9 ± 2.2 Women: 13.8 ± 2.2</li><li>70–87 Men: 13.2 ± 1.6 Women: 10.5 ± 3.5</li></ul>

[a]Assessment free at time of publication

Data from Functional Reach Test/Modified Functional Reach Test. (2013, December 4). *Shirley Ryan AbilityLab*. https://www.sralab.org/rehabilitation-measures/functional-reach-test-modified-functional-reach-test

Berg-Balance-Scale

1. SITTING TO STANDING
INSTRUCTIONS: Please stand up. Try not to use your hand for support.
( ) 4   able to stand without using hands and stabilize independently
( ) 3   able to stand independently using hands
( ) 2   able to stand using hands after several tries
( ) 1   needs minimal aid to stand or stabilize
( ) 0   needs moderate or maximal assistance to stand

2. STANDING UNSUPPORTED
INSTRUCTIONS: Please stand for 2 minutes without holding on.
( ) 4   able to stand safely for 2 minutes
( ) 3   able to stand 2 minutes with supervision
( ) 2   able to stand 30 seconds unsupported
( ) 1   needs several tries to stand 30 seconds unsupported
( ) 0   unable to stand 30 seconds unsupported

If a subject is able to stand 2 minutes unsupported, score full points for sitting unsupported. Proceed to item #4.

3. SITTING WITH BACK UNSUPPORTED BUT FEET SUPPORTED ON FLOOR OR ON A STOOL
INSTRUCTIONS: Please sit with arms folded for 2 minutes.
( ) 4   able to sit safely and securely for 2 minutes
( ) 3   able to sit 2 minutes under supervision
( ) 2   able to able to sit 30 seconds
( ) 1   able to sit 10 seconds
( ) 0   unable to sit without support 10 seconds

4. STANDING TO SITTING
INSTRUCTIONS: Please sit down.
( ) 4   sits safely with minimal use of hands
( ) 3   controls descent by using hands
( ) 2   uses back of legs against chair to control descent
( ) 1   sits independently but has uncontrolled descent
( ) 0   needs assistance to sit

5. TRANSFERS
INSTRUCTIONS: Arrange chair(s) for pivot transfer. Ask subject to transfer one way toward a seat with armrests and one way toward a seat without armrests. You may use two chairs (one with and one without armrests) or a bed and a chair.
( ) 4   able to transfer safely with minor use of hands
( ) 3   able to transfer safely definite need of hands
( ) 2   able to transfer with verbal cuing and/or supervision
( ) 1   needs one person to assistance
( ) 0   needs two people to assistance or supervise to be safe

6. STANDING UNSUPPORTED WITH EYES CLOSED
INSTRUCTIONS: Please close your eyes and stand still for 10 seconds.
( ) 4   able to stand 10 seconds safely
( ) 3   able to stand 10 seconds with supervision
( ) 2   able to stand 3 seconds
( ) 1   unable to keep eyes closed 3 seconds but stays safely
( ) 0   needs help to keep from falling

Berg-Balance-Scale continued......

7. STANDING UNSUPPORTED WITH FEET TOGETHER
INSTRUCTIONS: Place your feet together and stand without
holding on.
( ) 4   able to place feet together independently and stand
          1 minute safely
( ) 3   able to place feet together independently and stand
          1 minute with supervision
( ) 2   able to place feet together independently but unable
          to hold for 30 seconds
( ) 1   needs help to attain position but able to stand 15 seconds
          feet together
( ) 0   needs help to attain position and unable to hold for
          15 seconds

8. REACHING FORWARD WITH OUTSTRETCHED ARM WHILE STANDING
INSTRUCTIONS: Lift arm to 90 degrees. Stretch out your fingers and reach forward as far
as you can. (Examiner places a ruler at the end of fingertips when arm is at 90 degrees.
Fingers should not touch the ruler while reaching forward. The recorded measure is the
distance forward that the fingers reach while the subject is in the most forward lean position.
When possible, ask subject to use both arms when reaching to avoid rotation of the trunk.)
( ) 4   can reach forward confidently 25 cm (10 inches)
( ) 3   can reach forward 12 cm (5 inches)
( ) 2   can reach forward 5 cm (2 inches)
( ) 1   reaches forward but needs supervision
( ) 0   loses balance while trying/requires external support

9. PICK UP OBJECT FROM THE FLOOR FROM A STANDING POSITION
INSTRUCTIONS: Pick up the shoe/slipper, which is place in front of your feet.
( ) 4   able to pick up slipper safely and easily
( ) 3   able to pick up slipper but needs supervision
( ) 2   unable to pick up but reaches 2–5 cm(1–2 inches) from
          slipper and keeps balance independently
( ) 1   unable to pick up and needs supervision while trying
( ) 0   unable to try/needs assistance to keep from losing
          balance or falling

10. TURNING TO LOOK BEHIND OVER LEFT AND RIGHT SHOULDERS WHILE STANDING
INSTRUCTIONS: Turn to look directly behind you over toward the left shoulder. Repeat to the
right. Examiner may pick an object to look at directly behind the subject to encourage a
better twist turn.
( ) 4   looks behind from both sides and weight shifts well
( ) 3   looks behind one side only other side shows less weight
          shift
( ) 2   turns sideways only but maintains balance
( ) 1   needs supervision when turning
( ) 0   needs assistance to keep from losing balance or falling

Berg-Balance-Scale continued......

11. TURN 360 DEGREES

INSTRUCTIONS: Turn completely around in a full circle. Pause. Then turn a full circle in the other direction.

( ) 4   able to turn 360 degrees safely in 4 seconds or less
( ) 3   able to turn 360 degrees safely one side only
         4 seconds or less
( ) 2   able to turn 360 degrees safely but slowly
( ) 1   needs close supervision or verbal cuing
( ) 0   needs assistance while turning

12. PLACE ALTERNATE FOOT ON STEP OR STOOL WHILE STANDING UNSUPPORTED

INSTRUCTIONS: Place each foot alternately on the step/stool.
Continue until each foot has touch the step/stool four times.

( ) 4   able to stand independently and safely and complete
         8 steps in 20 seconds
( ) 3   able to stand independently and complete 8 steps in
         > 20 seconds
( ) 2   able to complete 4 steps without aid with supervision
( ) 1   able to complete > 2 steps needs minimal assistance
( ) 0   needs assistance to keep from falling/unable to try

13. STANDING UNSUPPORTED ONE FOOT IN FRONT

INSTRUCTIONS: (DEMONSTRATE TO SUBJECT) Place one foot directly in front of the other. If you feel that you cannot place your foot directly in front, try to step far enough ahead that the heel of your forward foot is ahead of the toes of the other foot. (To score 3 points, the length of the step should exceed the length of the other foot and the width of the stance should approximate the subject's normal stride width.)

( ) 4   able to place foot tandem independently and hold 30 seconds
( ) 3   able to place foot ahead independently and hold 30 seconds
( ) 2   able to take small step independently and hold 30 seconds
( ) 1   needs help to step but can hold 15 seconds
( ) 0   loses balance while stepping or standing

14. STANDING ON ONE LEG

INSTRUCTIONS: Stand on one leg as long as you can without holding on

( ) 4   able to lift leg independently and hold > 10 seconds
( ) 3   able to lift leg independently and hold 5–10 seconds
( ) 2   able to lift leg independently and hold $\geq$ 3 seconds
( ) 1   tries to lift leg unable to hold 3 seconds but remains
         standing independently
( ) 0   unable to try of needs assistance to prevent fall

( )   TOTAL SCORE (Maximum = 56)

Berg-Balance-Scale

Name: _____   Date: _____

Location: _____   Rater: _____

ITEM DESCRIPTION	SCORE (0–4)
1. Sitting to standing	_____
2. Standing unsupported	_____
3. Sitting unsupported	_____
4. Standing to sitting	_____
5. Transfers	_____
6. Standing with eyes closed	_____
7. Standing with feet together	_____
8. Reaching forward with outstretched arm	_____
9. Retrieving object from floor	_____
10. Turning to look behind	_____
11. Turning 360 degrees	_____
12. Placing alternate foot on stool	_____
13. Standing with one foot in front	_____
14. Standing on one foot	_____
Total	_____

GENERAL INSTRUCTIONS

Please document each task and/or give instructions as written. When scoring, please
record the lowest response category that applies for each item.

In most items, the subject is asked to maintain a given position for a specific time.
Progressively more points are deducted if:

- The time or distance requirements are not met
- The subject's performance warrants supervision
- The subject touches an external support or receives assistance
  from the examiner

Subject should understand that they must maintain their balance while attempting the tasks.
The choices of which leg to stand on or how far to reach are left to the subject. Poor
judgment will adversely influence the performance and the scoring.

Equipment required for testing is a stopwatch or watch with a second hand, and a ruler or
other indicator of 2, 5, and 10 inches. Chairs used during testing should be a reasonable
height. Either a step or a stool of average step height may be used for item # 12.

Functional Assessments

PURPOSE	FEATURES	TIME	INTERPRETATION OF SCORES
BARTHEL INDEX (BI) (Free[a])			
An ordinal scale that assesses performance of basic activities of daily living (BADLs) and mobility related activities of daily living (MR-ADLs) and estimates level of assistance required/caregiver burden.	Performance-based assessment of 10 domains, including feeding, bathing, dressing, grooming, bowel and bladder control, toilet use, transfers, mobility, and stairs.	30–45 min	• 80–100: Likely appropriate for independent living • 60–79: Minimally dependent • 40–59: Moderately dependent • 20–39: Very dependent • <20: Total dependency

Data from Barthel Index. (2020, May 21). *Shirley Ryan AbilityLab*. https://www.sralab.org/rehabilitation-measures/barthel-index

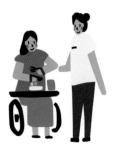

THE CANADIAN OCCUPATIONAL PERFORMANCE MEASURE (COPM)

A client-centered evaluation focusing on areas of self-care, productivity, and leisure as perceived by the patient.	Occupational therapist (OT) conducts a semi-structured interview that may include direct observation in order to identify problem areas. Next, the patient uses a 10-point scale to rate her own level of performance and satisfaction with performance.	15–30 min	• Designed as an outcome measure instead of a norm-referenced evaluation, scores are compared only against previous scores (such as time of eval to reassessment). • A change of at least two points is considered clinically important.

Data from Canadian Occupational Performance Measure. (2019, June 1). *Shirley Ryan AbilityLab*. https://www.sralab.org/rehabilitation-measures/canadian-occupational-performance-measure

FUNCTIONAL INDEPENDENCE MEASURE (FIM)

An outcome measure often used for data collection and reporting. Assesses level of disability based on evaluation of functional performance and cognition.	Performance-based assessment of 18 domains: 13 ADLs/MR-ADLs and 5 cognitive components.	30–45 min	• Each task is rated from 1 (total assistance) to 7 (completely independent). • It is intended to be administered at admission, reassessment, and discharge for the purpose of quantifying changes in functional status.

Data from Functional Independence Measure (FIM). (n.d.). *Physiopedia*. Retrieved September 5, 2021, from https://www.physio-pedia.com/Functional_Independence _Measure_(FIM)

PURPOSE	FEATURES	TIME	INTERPRETATION OF SCORES
KATZ INDEX OF INDEPENDENCE IN ACTIVITIES OF DAILY LIVING (KATZ) (Free[a])			
A basic tool that assesses functional status and transfer ability.	OT may observe patient performance or interview patient to assess level of function in areas of bathing, dressing, toileting, transferring, continence, and feeding. One point assigned for each category in which patient is independent.	5–30 min	• 6 points indicate full function. • 3–5 points indicate moderate impairment. • 2 points or less indicate severe functional impairment.

Data from Katz Index of Independence in Activities of Daily Living. (2016, December 1). *Shirley Ryan AbilityLab*. https://www.sralab.org/rehabilitation-measures/katz-index-independence-activities-daily-living

PURPOSE	FEATURES	TIME	INTERPRETATION OF SCORES
KOHLMAN EVALUATION OF LIVING SKILLS (KELS)			
A comprehensive evaluation to determine appropriateness of independent living for patients with physical and/ or cognitive disability.	OT may observe patient performance or interview patient regarding 17 basic skills that are assessed within the five domains of self-care, safety/ health, money management, transportation, telephone, work, and leisure.	20–60 min	• 0–5.5 points indicate patient is likely able to live independently. • 6–17 points indicate inability to live independently without assistance.

Data from Kohlman Evaluation of Living Skills. (2019, April 26). *Shirley Ryan* Ability-Lab.https://www.sralab.org/rehabilitation-measures/kohlman-evaluation-living-skills

ASSESSMENT

PURPOSE	FEATURES	TIME	INTERPRETATION OF SCORES
LAWTON INSTRUMENTAL ACTIVITIES OF DAILY LIVING (IADLs) SCALE (Free[a])			
An eight-item questionnaire that assesses higher level skills required to live in an independent setting.	Eight domains of function assessed by means of self-report including ability to use telephone, shopping, food prep, housekeeping, laundry, transportation, medication management, and finances.	10–15 min	• Score ranges from 0 to 8 with a lower score indicating higher level of dependence.

Data from Graf, C. G. (2008, April). *Lawton—Brody Instrumental Activities of Daily Living Scale (I.A.D.L.).* Alz.Org. https://www.alz.org/careplanning/downloads/lawton-iadl.pdf

PERFORMANCE ASSESSMENT OF SELF-CARE SKILLS (PASS) (Free[a])			
A comprehensive, client-centered evaluation focusing on person, environment, and occupation to determine appropriateness of independent living.	Performance-based assessment of four domains (functional mobility, self-care, cognitive-based IADLs, and physical-based IADLs) that consist of 26 core tasks. Patient is rated on level of independence, safety, and adequacy for each task.	1.5–3 h	• Extensive normative data available by impairment/ condition accessible online.

[a]Assessment free at time of publication.
Data from Performance Assessment of Self-Care Skills. (2015, June 5). *Shirley Ryan AbilityLab.* https://www.sralab.org/rehabilitationmeasures/performance-assessment-self-care-skills

THE BARTHEL INDEX	Patient Name: _____	
	Rater Name: _____	
	Date: _____	

Activity	Score

FEEDING
    0 = unable
    5 = needs help cutting, spreading butter, etc., or requires modified diet
    10 = independent   _____

BATHING
    0 = dependent
    5 = independent (or in shower)   _____

GROOMING
    0 = needs help with personal care
    5 = independent face/hair/teeth/shaving (implements provided)   _____

DRESSING
    0 = dependent
    5 = needs help but can do about half unaided
    10 = independent (including buttons, zips, laces, etc.)   _____

BOWELS
    0 = incontinent (or needs to be given enemas)
    5 = occasional accident
    10 = continent   _____

BLADDER
    0 = incontinent, or catheterized and
    unable to manage alone
    5 = occasional accident
    10 = continent   _____

TOILET USE
    0 = dependent
    5 = needs some help, but can do something alone
    10 = independent (on and off, dressing, wiping)   _____

TRANSFERS (BED TO CHAIR AND BACK)
    0 = unable, no sitting balance
    5 = major help (one or two people, physical), can sit
    10 = minor help (verbal or physical)
    15 = independent   _____

MOBILITY (ON LEVEL SURFACES)
    0 = immobile or < 50 yards
    5 = wheelchair independent, including corners, > 50 yards
    10 = walks with help of one person (verbal or physical) > 50 yards
    15 = independent (but may use any aid; for example, stick) > 50 yards   _____

STAIRS
    0 = unable
    5 = needs help (verbal, physical, carrying aid)
    10 = independent   _____

TOTAL (0–100):   _____

Adapted from Mahoney FI, Barthel D. "Functional evaluation: the Barthel Index." *Maryland State Med Journal* 1965;14:56-61.

ASSESSMENT

12

Cognitive Assessments

PURPOSE	FEATURES	TIME	INTERPRETATION OF SCORE
MONTREAL COGNITIVE ASSESSMENT (MOCA)			
Detects mild cognitive impairment	Pen-and-paper test of short-term memory, visuospatial ability, attention, concentration, orientation, language, and abstract reasoning.	10 min	• ≥26 indicates normal cognitive function • <26 indicates potential cognitive impairment

Data from MoCA—Cognitive Assessment. (n.d.). *MoCA—Cognitive Assessment*. Retrieved September 5, 2021, from https://www.mocatest.org/

PURPOSE	FEATURES	TIME	INTERPRETATION OF SCORE
GLASGOW COMA SCALE (GCS) (Free[a])			
Neurological scale used to document level of consciousness	Three components are assessed including "eyes," "motor," and "verbal"	<5 min	• Eyes are scored 1–4 with scores ranging from not opening eyes (1), to opens eyes spontaneously (4). • Verbal ranges from (1) makes no sound to (5) oriented, converses normally. • Motor score ranges from makes no movements (1) to obeys commands (6). • Results are recorded as (example) GCS 9 = E3 V2 M4 at 16:45.

Data from Jain, S. (2021, June 20). *Glasgow Coma Scale—StatPearls—NCBI Bookshelf*. NCBI. https://www.ncbi.nlm.nih.gov/books/NBK513298/

PURPOSE	FEATURES	TIME	INTERPRETATION OF SCORE
MINI MENTAL STATE EXAM (MMSE) (Free[a])			
Detects mild cognitive impairment and assesses cognitive changes over time	Pen-and-paper test of orientation, attention, memory, language, delayed recall, and visuospatial cognition.	5–10 min	• ≥24 indicates normal cognitive function • 19–23 indicates mild cognitive impairment • 10–18 indicates moderate cognitive impairment • ≤9 indicates severe cognitive impairment

Data from Oxford Medical Education (2016, April 15). *Mini-mental state examination (MMSE)*. Oxford Medical Education. https://oxfordmedicaleducation.com/geriatrics/mini-mental-state-examination-mmse/

RANCHO LOS AMIGOS SCALE (RLAS) (Free[a])			
An 8-point scale used to evaluate cognitive functioning and track progress with therapy post traumatic brain injury (TBI)	Cognitive level is assessed based on observation of behavioral patterns. Classification helps guide plan of care and provides standardized communication for the care team. A family guide to the eight levels also provides techniques on caring for the patient.	NA	• Level 1: No response • Level 2: Generalized response • Level 3: Localized response • Level 4: Confused agitated • Level 5: Confused agitated, inappropriate • Level 6: Confused appropriate • Level 7: Automatic appropriate • Level 8: Purposeful appropriate

Data from Lin, K. (2020, August 30). *Ranchos Los Amigos—StatPearls—NCBI Bookshelf*. NCBI. https://www.ncbi.nlm.nih.gov/books/NBK448151/

ASSESSMENT

PURPOSE	FEATURES	TIME	INTERPRETATION OF SCORE
ALLEN COGNITIVE LEVEL SCREEN (ACLS)			
Scores are used to provide an estimate of abilities and determine appropriateness for independent living	Learning potential and problem solving assessed. Leather lacing tool used to learn and demonstrate three stitching tasks of increasing complexity. Performance based.	20 min	1. Highly impaired cognition 2. Dependent 3. Supervision and cues 4. May live independently with established routines and frequent checks 5. Minimal community support or occasional checks 6. Intact cognition, able to plan for the future

Data from Home. (2021, January 7). *Allen Cognitive Level Screen Assessment.* https://allencognitive.com/

SAINT LOUIS UNIVERSITY MENTAL STATUS EXAMINATION (SLUMS) (Free[a])			
Detects mild cognitive impairment	Pen-and-paper test of short-term memory/delayed recall, orientation, basic math, word retrieval, attention, and visuospatial awareness.	5–10 min	• 27–30 is considered normal for a patient with a high school education • >25 is considered normal for patients with less than a high school education • 21–26 suggests a mild neurocognitive disorder • 0–20 indicates dementia

[a]Assessment free at time of evaluation
Data from Saint Louis University Mental Status Exam. (2019, May 15). *Shirley Ryan AbilityLab.* https://www.sralab.org/rehabilitation-measures/saint-louis-university-mental-status-exam

VAMC
SLUMS EXAMINATION

Questions about this assessment tool? E-mail aging@slu.edu

Name_____ Age _____

Is the patient alert? _____ Level of education _____

__/1 ❶ 1. What day of the week is it?

__/1 ❶ 2. What is the year?

__/1 ❶ 3. What state are we in?

4. Please remember these five objects. I will ask you what they are later.
   Apple   Pen   Tie   House   Car

5. You have $100 and you go to the store and buy a dozen apples for $3 and a tricycle for $20.
   ❶ How much did you spend?
   ❷ How much do you have left?

__/3

6. Please name as many animals as you can in one minute.

__/3   ❶ 0–4 animals   ❶ 5–9 animals   ❷ 10–14 animals   ❸ 15+ animals

__/5 7. What were the five objects I asked you to remember? 1 point for each one correct.

8. I am going to give you a series of numbers and I would like you to give them to me
   backwards. For example, if I say 42, you would say 24.

__/2   ❶ 87   ❶ 648   ❶ 8537

9. This is a clock face. Please put in the hour markers and the time at
   ten minutes to eleven o'clock.

❷ Hour markers okay

__/4 ❷ Time correct

❶ 10. Please place an X in the triangle.

❶ Which of the above figures is largest?

__/2

11. I am going to tell you a story. Please listen carefully because afterwards, I'm going to ask
    you some questions about it.

Jill was a very successful stockbroker. She made a lot of money on the stock market. She then met
Jack, a devastatingly handsome man. She married him and had three children. They lived in Chicago.
She then stopped work and stayed at home to bring up her children. When they were teenagers, she
went back to work. She and Jack lived happily ever after.

❷ What was the female's name?   ❷ What work did she do?

__/8 ❷ When did she go back to work?   ❷ What state did she live in?

_____ TOTAL SCORE

SCORING	
HIGH SCHOOL EDUCATION	**LESS THAN HIGH SCHOOL EDUCATION**
27–30 .... NORMAL 25–30
21–26 .... MILD NEUROCOGNITIVE DISORDER 20–24
1–20 .... DEMENTIA 1–19

_____   _____   _____
CLINICIAN'S SIGNATURE   **DATE**   **TIME**

SH Tariq, N Tumosa, JT Chibnall, HM Perry III, and JE Morley. The Saint Louis University Mental Status (SLUMS)
Examination for detecting mild cognitive impairment and dementia is more sensitive than the Mini-Mental Status
Examination (MMSE) - A pilot study. *Am J Geriatr Psych* 14:900-10, 2006.

13

Home Safety Eval/ Checklist

Specific recommendations will depend on a variety of issues, such as the patient's particular deficits, functional level, financial means, family or community support to assist with implementing changes, and the permission to make such changes if the patient is not the homeowner.

COMMON AREAS

- Furniture is arranged to allow for safe mobility throughout home.
- Couches and chairs are of suitable height and design.
  - Recommend risers, couch cane, or alternative seating if too low or if lacking arms, for ease of transfer.
  - Recommend removal of unsafe furniture such as swivel chairs.
- All throw rugs have been removed or secured.
- Pathways are clear of clutter, cords, or other trip hazards.
- Lighting is sufficient throughout home with easily accessible light switches.
- Working smoke detectors are present throughout home with at least one carbon monoxide detector on each floor.

KITCHEN

- All items are within reach to avoid use of footstool.
- Towels, napkins, and other flammables are not stored on or near stovetop.
- Cleaning agents are easily identifiable and stored separate from food.
- Auto shut-off features present if appropriate.
- Lighting is sufficient with easily accessible light switches.

BEDROOM

- Furniture is arranged to allow for safe mobility.
- Light switch and phone are accessible by bedside.
- Bed assist bar present for safety of bed transfer if appropriate.
- All throw rugs have been removed or secured.
- Bed is of proper height.
- Frequently used items in closet are easily accessible.
- Lighting is sufficient.

BATHROOM

- Adaptive equipment installed for safe toilet transfer, such as riser, raised toilet seat, safety frame, or mounted grab bar, if appropriate.
- Adaptive equipment installed for safe bathing and shower transfer, such as shower chair or transfer bench, grab bars at entrance to and inside shower, handheld shower head, and nonslip mat on tub/shower floor, if appropriate.
- Removal of sliding shower doors, if appropraite, to be replaced by rod and curtain, allowing more space for transfer or use of transfer bench.
- Throw rugs have been removed and replaced with rubber-backed mats or secured with double-sided tape.
- Lighting is sufficient with easily accessible light switches.

STAIRS

- Nonskid strips installed for traction if stairs are not carpeted.
- At least one handrail present that extends the length of the stairs (installed 34–38 inches above the floor).
- Use of contrast tape or accent paint if patient has low vision.
- Lighting is sufficient with easily accessible light switches.

GARAGE

- All clutter or tripping hazards have been removed.
- Recommend repair of any uneven or cracked cement.
- Any raised thresholds have been marked with contrast tape or accent paint.
- Lighting is sufficient with easily accessible light switches.

ASSESSMENT

ENTRANCE TO HOME

- Handrails present next to all stairs (installed 34–38 inches above the floor).
- Grab bar installed next to door (approximately 36 inches from the ground), if appropriate.
- Yard maintained (bushes trimmed, overgrown ground cover removed, etc.) for clear pathway to front door.
- Ramp present for wheelchair entry if appropriate (length should be 1 foot for every inch of rise).
- Recommend repair of any uneven or cracked cement.
- Lighting is sufficient with easily accessible light switches.

OTHER

- Recommend medical alert system, if appropriate. If patient declines suggestion, recommend keeping cell phone within reach at all times.
- Removal of any expired prescription/over-the-counter medications.
- Recommend double-sided tape or rubber rug pad to secure rugs if patient declines removal.
- Check status of CO_2/smoke detectors.

14

Underlying Dysfunction

UNDERLYING DYSFUNCTION

The following list can be referred to during an observational assessment of occupational performance in order to identify underlying impairments. Establishing the link between a decline in occupational performance and specific impairments can help guide treatment planning as well as demonstrate the need for skilled occupational therapy (OT) intervention in documentation.

COGNITIVE SKILLS

- Problem solving
- Planning
- Learning ability
- Comprehension
- Attention
- Memory
- Sequencing
- Reasoning
- Judgment
- Orientation

NEUROMUSCULOSKELETAL/MOTOR AND PRAXIS SKILLS

- Muscle strength and tone
- Range of motion and joint stability
- Gross and fine motor coordination
- Sitting and standing postural stability
- Balance
- Gait pattern
- Endurance and activity tolerance
- Praxis: Ideation → motor planning → execution → feedback/adaptation.

SENSORY FUNCTIONS

- Visual
- Hearing
- Tactile
- Vestibular
- Proprioceptive
- Pain

SENSORY-PERCEPTUAL SKILLS

Auditory perceptual skills:
- Auditory awareness
- Auditory discrimination
- Auditory identification
- Auditory comprehension

Visual perceptual skills:
- Visual discrimination
- Form constancy
- Visual memory
- Visual sequential memory
- Visual closure
- Visual spatial relations
- Visual figure ground

Tactile perceptual skills:
- Stereognosis/haptic perception

PROCESS SKILLS

- The ability to effectively carry out an activity, using tools if necessary, and adjusting performance if difficulties arise.
  - Initiates, continues, and terminates the task
  - Paces, organizes, and sequences the task
  - Chooses and uses tools appropriately
  - Attends to task, seeking information when needed, and adjusts performance to be effective

EMOTIONAL REGULATION SKILLS

- Self-awareness
- Inhibition/impulse control
- Mental flexibility
- Coping mechanisms
- Appropriate responses

COMMUNICATION AND SOCIAL INTERACTION SKILLS

- To cooperate within a group setting and adhere to established norms.
- To effectively interact and communicate via language, actions, and behaviors.

Adapted from *Occupational Therapy Practice Framework: Domain and Process—Fourth Edition* | *American Journal of Occupational Therapy*. (2020, August 1). AJOT. https://ajot.aota.org/article.aspx?articleid=2766507

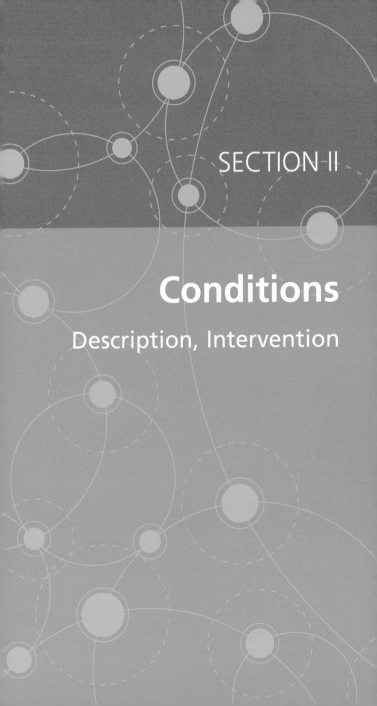

SECTION II

Conditions
Description, Intervention

15

Aftercare Following Joint Replacement

AFTERCARE FOLLOWING JOINT REPLACEMENT

Arthroplasty (joint replacement) is a surgical procedure that involves removal of old cartilage, resurfacing of the bones, and placement of a prosthesis (artificial joint). Symptomatic osteoarthritis is the most common indication for surgery (Ferguson et al., 2018). Given the restorative nature of joint replacements, patients generally experience improvements in occupational performance and overall quality of life.

ASSESSMENT

Ensure adherence to all precautions during assessments.

Basic:
- Range of motion (ROM)
- Manual muscle testing (MMT)
  - *ROM and strength of affected joint to be assessed once permitted*

Functional:
- Modified Barthel Index (MBI)
- Functional Independence Measure (FIM)
- Lawton Instrumental Activities of Daily Living (IADL) Scale

Balance:
- Berg Balance Scale (BBS)

Pain:
- Verbal Rating Scale
- 0–10 Numeric Pain Intensity Scale
- Wong Baker Faces Scale
- Brief Pain Inventory

CONDITIONS

INTERVENTION
TOTAL SHOULDER REPLACEMENT/HEMIARTHROPLASTY/TSA

- A comprehensive shoulder protocol is beyond the scope of this pocketbook but should be followed as set forth (or approved) by the referring surgeon for optimal healing. **Generally, this includes a period of passive range of motion (PROM) for approximately 2–3 weeks, followed by active range of motion (AROM), and finally resistive exercises.** Treatment progression is based on multiple factors, including but not limited to the specific surgical approach, any postoperative complications, and the individual progress of each patient.
- **Sling should be worn continuously for 3–4 weeks** unless bathing, dressing, or performing AROM below shoulder.
- **No AROM of shoulder initially**, but daily AROM below shoulder (elbow, wrist, and hand) is important to avoid stiffness/contractures.
- **No lifting, pushing, or pulling, initially**. After approximately 3–4 weeks, light lifting (no greater than a coffee cup) is typically allowed.
- In supine, **a small pillow or towel roll should be placed behind the elbow (not shoulder)** to avoid shoulder hyperextension or anterior capsular stretch.
- Instruct in completing transfers **without pushing up or lowering down on affected upper extremity**.
- **Edema** of hand can be controlled using **retrograde massage, compression glove, and fist pumps or ball squeezes. Arm can be elevated above level of heart** once patient is cleared to do so following the protocol.
- **Educate in hemi-dressing techniques** such as when donning shirt, the affected upper extremity (UE) should be placed in sleeve first, but when doffing shirt, affected UE should come out last, and/or recommend modified upper body clothing.
- Once out of sling, **educate in compensatory strategies to avoid internal rotation and adduction together with extension** that occurs when reaching behind back for bathroom hygiene or to tuck in shirt.
- The affected side will likely remain in a sling for at least 3–4 weeks, thus **assessing dexterity of the unaffected**

upper extremity during ADL performance is also important in order to guide specific intervention during the healing phase.

JOINT PROTECTION OF REVERSE TOTAL SHOULDER REPLACEMENT/R-TSA

- **The same precautions as a conventional total shoulder apply;** however, there is a higher occurrence of joint dislocation following reverse total shoulder, with the most provoking combination being in the above-mentioned position of **internal rotation and adduction together with extension**. As such, it is imperative that patients are **educated in compensatory techniques for all activities of daily living (ADLs) that require reaching behind the back**. Additionally, PROM into shoulder internal rotation is generally avoided until 6 weeks post op.

TOTAL HIP ARTHROPLASTY/THA

- **ADL retraining to integrate hip precautions** for approximately 6–8 weeks while joint heals.
- Utilization of **adaptive equipment** can help patients adhere to the following precautions. Common useful equipment includes dressing stick, sock aid, long-handled shoehorn, shower chair, and riser for toilet.
  - POSTERIOR APPROACH
    - **No hip flexion greater than 90 degrees.**
    - **No adduction beyond midline.**
    - **No internal rotation.**
    - **Generally observed for 6–8 weeks.**
  - ANTERIOR APPROACH
    - **No hip extension.**
    - **No abduction.**
    - **No adduction beyond midline.**
    - **No external rotation.**
    - **Generally observed for 6–8 weeks.**

TOTAL KNEE ARTHROPLASTY/TKA

- **ADL retraining to integrate knee precautions** for approximately 6–8 weeks while joint heals
  - No rolled-up towel or pillow behind knee.

CONDITIONS

- No kneeling.
- Do not torque/twist knee.

Occupation-based intervention/ADL retraining examples:

- A patient in the acute stage of recovery from a right total shoulder arthroplasty (R TSA) is seen for her morning ADL routine. Beginning with upper body dressing, the patient is instructed to lay a loose-fitting shirt, front side down, on her lap. The occupational therapist (OT) educates the patient in proper sequencing including placing affected UE through sleeve first followed by the unaffected side. The patient is then directed to pull the shirt over her head with the unaffected UE and the sling is replaced by the OT. The patient is given verbal cues to sit on the edge of bed to don pants due to poor+ static standing balance. The OT demonstrates holding the center of the elastic waistband and bending down to thread each foot through the pant leg. The patient returns demonstration requiring minimal assist to complete the task. She is then instructed to lay supine and bridge hips in order to hike pants over hips using unaffected UE only. She is verbally cued to perform hygiene and grooming tasks with left/unaffected UE in sitting. Following a bowel movement she struggles to perform peri-care with toilet paper using the nondominant left hand. The OT provides wet wipes and trains patient in single leg lift using small stool for increased access to perineal area. The OT also recommends attachable bidet to be installed on her toilet at home.
- Following left total hip arthroplasty (L THA), a patient is instructed in lower body dressing with the use of adaptive equipment while seated in his wheelchair. The OT demonstrates how to use a long-handled reacher to hook the waist band and lower the pants down to the foot of the operated left lower extremity (L LE), which is threaded through the pant leg first. The OT verbally emphasizes the importance of proper sequencing in order to reduce strain on the operated LE as the second step of threading the remaining unoperated R LE is demonstrated. The OT also demonstrates how the reacher eliminates the need to lean forward in order to adhere to the hip flexion precaution. Patient is given verbal cues to extend the operated LE out in front prior to standing in order to widen the hip angle

and maintain the hip flexion precaution. He stands to hike pants over hips and is cued to keep the operated LE extended when returning to a seated position. The OT then demonstrates the use of a sock aid to don socks. The patient returns demonstration requiring verbal cues to drop the sock aid to his feet rather than leaning down. Lastly, the OT demonstrates the use of a long-handled shoehorn to don shoes. The patient performs the action while maintaining all precautions.

OTHER CONSIDERATIONS

- **Ice 4–5 times per day** for 15–20 minutes for pain management.
- OT to **endorse ambulation device** as prescribed by PT following hip and knee surgery.

PROVIDING CLIENT-CENTERED CARE:

- As joint replacements generally bring about only a temporary decrease in independence, patients may prefer to enlist the help of a caregiver (e.g., a spouse, professional attendant, etc.) during the healing phase rather than learning compensatory strategies or buying adaptive equipment. Additionally, patients may require assistance with ADLs at baseline and thus prefer to focus on other activities. In either case, caregiver training should be provided to ensure proper handling of the affected extremity. A thorough interview at time of evaluation will help to determine preferences and baseline performance in order to create a plan of care that reflects the patient's preferences.

CONDITIONS

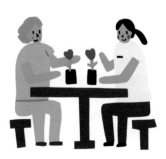

16

Alzheimer Disease/ Dementia

ALZHEIMER DISEASE/DEMENTIA

Alzheimer disease (AD) is a progressive disorder characterized by an insidious decline of cognitive and physical functioning that eventually leads to severe impairment (Aisen et al., 2017). These degenerative changes are the result of beta-amyloid plaques and neurofibrillary tangles made from tau proteins that cause damage to neurons and synapses. Dementia, on the other hand, is not a specific disease, rather, a decline of cognitive functioning brought about by various causes such as AD, Lewy bodies, vascular disease, drugs, and alcohol (Lopez & Kuller, 2019).

ASSESSMENT

Cognitive function/screening for dementia:

- Mini Mental State Exam (MMSE)
- Montreal Cognitive Assessment (MoCA)
- Clock Drawing Test
- Saint Louis University Mental Status Examination (SLUMS)
- AD8 Dementia Screening Interview

Progression of disease & staging:

- Functional Assessment Staging Test (FAST)
- Clinicians Global Impression of Change

Functional ability & mobility:

- Modified Barthel Index (MBI)

- Functional Independence Measure (FIM)
- Lawton Instrumental Activities of Daily Living (IADL) Scale
- Timed Up and Go Test (TUG)
- Five Times Sit to Stand

Balance & fall risk:
- Berg Balance Scale (BBS)
- Tinetti Balance and Gait Assessment
- Modified Clinical Test of Sensory Interaction in Balance (CTSIB-M)

Ability to live independently:
- Allen Cognitive Level Screen (ACLS)
- Kohlman Evaluation of Living Skills (KELS)

Depression:
- The Geriatric Depression Scale (GDS)

Behavior:
- Neuropsychiatric Inventory

Quality of life:
- AD-related Quality of Life Scale (QoL-AD)

ASSESSING DEMENTIA-RELATED BEHAVIORS:

Problematic behaviors are often a form of communication and may be related to an underlying issue, such as

- **Environmental:**
  - Changes to personal living space
  - Competing stimuli
- **Physiological:**
  - Pain, discomfort, illness, infection
  - Side effects of medication
- **Psychological:**
  - Frustration with inability to communicate needs effectively
  - Loneliness

CONDITIONS

- **Task related:**
  - Demand that exceeds ability
- **Change related:**
  - Changes in schedule, routine, caregiver, etc.

NORMAL BEHAVIORAL RESPONSES TO STRESS		DEMENTIA-RELATED BEHAVIORAL RESPONSES TO STRESS
Engages in physical activity	→	Wanders/paces
Social outlets	→	Repeats the same question/ initiates conversation even if nonsensical
Bathes/showers, changes clothes	→	Doffs clothing
Goes shopping	→	Rummages and hoards
Engages in sexual activity	→	Displays sexually inappropriate behavior

Source: Weissberg, K. (2020, February). *Dementia Management: Techniques for Staging and Intervention* [Slides]. https://occupationaltherapy.com

INTERVENTION

MILD COGNITIVE IMPAIRMENT:

- **Spaced retrieval therapy:**
  - Eliciting the recall of information with progressively longer intervals.
- **Dual-task interventions:**
  - Working on two tasks simultaneously. This can be a physical and cognitive task, two cognitive tasks, or two physical tasks concurrently.
- **Errorless learning:**
  - The use of multimodal cues to prevent mistakes when relearning a task.
- Recommend **memory aids** such as a calendar, planner, whiteboard, and sticky notes.
- Guide patient and caregiver in **establishing a daily routine** in order to create predictability and reduce anxiety.
- Provide **three-step cueing max** at one time and focus on the whole task.

Occupation-based intervention/activity of daily living (ADL) retraining examples:

- Employing the principles of dual task intervention, the patient is asked to switch between creating a grocery list and standing to fold laundry.

- Utilizing the errorless learning technique, a patient is guided through a supervised bathing activity with use of verbal and visual cues to prevent any mistakes from occurring throughout the session.

MODERATE COGNITIVE IMPAIRMENT:

- **Create signage** with appropriate font size and visual contrast.

- Recommend **memory aids** (see above).

- Guide patient and caregiver in **establishing a daily routine** in order to create predictability and reduce anxiety.

- Use **repetitive sequencing** to facilitate long-term learning.

- Provide **two-step cueing max** at one time and focus on the components of the task.

- **Reduce distractions.**

Occupation-based intervention/ADL retraining examples:

- The occupational therapist (OT) focuses exclusively on the steps to don a shirt, providing two-step verbal cues throughout the process. The OT breaks the activity into smaller steps by first focusing on retrieving the shirt from the closet. Next, the patient is cued to prepare by sitting and placing garment face down on her lap. The patient is then guided through the steps for donning and doffing. The patient is asked to repeat the same process three times in order to retain the dressing procedure (repetitive sequencing).

SEVERE COGNITIVE IMPAIRMENT:

- Focus on the **sensory aspects** of the activity.

- **Modify and adapt** the environment.

- Place attention on **residual abilities** rather than impairments.

CONDITIONS

- Establish/train caregivers in a **contracture management program**.

- Provide **one-step cueing max**.

Occupation-based intervention/ADL retraining examples:

- The patient and caregiver are trained in incorporating a contracture management program with self-care activities. For example, the patient's shirt is donned while performing shoulder flexion portion of the passive range of motion (PROM) program. OT then assists to facilitate teeth and hair brushing during shoulder external rotation.

- OT guides the patient in a basic seated cooking activity using five or less ingredients with a focus on the scent and texture of each ingredient.

OTHER CONSIDERATIONS

- **A thorough interview with a reliant informant** should be conducted as patients with AD are often poor historians.

- **The OT can determine and advise if a higher level of care or an alternative living situation with increased supervision is indicated.** As an objective measure, research demonstrates that the ACLS is quite accurate in determining a patient's functional level and appropriateness for independent living (McCraith, 2016).

- Various studies have established a link between physical activity and cognitive performance (Bherer et al., 2013). **Establishing an exercise program that includes an aerobic component** may help slow the progression of the disease as well as help to prevent falls. Ensure no duplication of services with physical therapy (PT).

- Falls with hip fracture are much higher in the cognitively impaired population (Dautel, 2019); thus, it is important to **address fall prevention** (see Education: Fall Prevention).

- The patient should be **assessed for depression** given the high prevalence in this population (*Alzheimer's disease facts and figures*, 2020).

- **Caregivers should be provided information regarding services** such as respite care, local or online support groups, and paid caregiver services.

PROVIDING CLIENT-CENTERED CARE:

- For patients with AD it is especially beneficial to utilize familiar occupations. For example, potting a plant would be an appropriate fine motor task for a patient who was an avid gardener. Interviewing a family member can help provide information regarding meaningful occupations and past interests/hobbies.

Alzheimer's disease facts and figures. (2020, March 1). Alzheimer's Association. https://alz-journals.onlinelibrary.wiley.com/doi/full/10.1002/alz.12068

17

Burns

BURNS			
CLASSIFICATION	TISSUE DEPTH	CHARACTERISTICS	HEALING TIME
Superficial (First-degree)	Superficial epidermis	Erythema (redness), blanching, no blistering, mild pain.	3–7 days
Superficial partial thickness (Superficial second-degree)	Epidermis, upper dermis	Erythema, blisters (wet if blisters have ruptured), pain, mild edema.	<14 days
Deep partial thickness (Deep second-degree)	Epidermis, majority of dermis	Erythema, large blisters (wet if blisters have ruptured), moderate edema, severe pain. Skin appendages for epithelial regeneration intact.	>14 days
Full thickness (Third-degree)	Epidermis and dermis	Pale, dry, hard skin. Nerve endings and skin appendages destroyed. Absent sensation of pain.	Months

BURNS			
CLASSIFICATION	TISSUE DEPTH	CHARACTERISTICS	HEALING TIME
Subdermal	Epidermis, dermis, and underlying structure (fat muscle, bone) involved	Charring, exposed fat and muscle tissue. Nerve endings and skin appendages destroyed. Absent sensation of pain. Surgical intervention required.	Possible amputation

Data from Pendleton, H., & Schultz-Krohn, W. (2017). *Pedretti's Occupational Therapy: Practice Skills for Physical Dysfunction (Occupational Therapy Skills for Physical Dysfunction (Pedretti))*. 8th ed. Mosby.

WOUND HEALING PHASES	
Inflammatory phase	Wound is painful, warm, red, and edematous. Neutrophils and monocytes arrive to debride the wound, clearing out bacteria and debris. Lasts 4–6 days.
Proliferation phase	Wound is less painful and becomes raised. Granulation (formation of new connective tissue and blood vessels) and re-epithelialization (formation of collagen over the wound bed) occur, contracting tissue to reduce size of wound. Lasts 4–24 days.
Maturation phase	Collagen remodeling softens and flattens wound. Lasts 21 days to 2 years.

RULE OF NINES		
Head	Rostral	4.5%
	Caudal	4.5%
Torso	Anterior	18%
	Posterior	18%
Right arm	Ventral	4.5%
	Dorsal	4.5%
Left arm	Ventral	4.5%
	Dorsal	4.5%
Right leg	Anterior	9%
	Posterior	9%
Left leg	Anterior	9%
	Posterior	9%
Genitalia/perineum	N/A	1%

Lewis et al. (2017).

ASSESSMENT

Prior to evaluation, conduct a thorough chart review for information regarding burn classification, total burn surface area (TBSA), location, joints involved, and evidence of smoke inhalation injury.

Full occupational therapy (OT) evaluations are generally postponed until after the emergent phase.

Basic:

- Range of motion (ROM)
- Manual muscle testing (MMT)
- Sensation
  - Semmes-Weinstein Monofilament Test (SWMT)

Functional Ability & Mobility:

- Modified Barthel Index (MBI)
- Functional Independence Measure (FIM)
- Canadian Occupational Performance Measure (COPM)
- Performance Assessment of Self-Care Skills (PASS)

Pain:

- Verbal Rating Scale
- 0–10 Numeric Pain Intensity Scale
- Wong Baker Faces Scale
- The Brief Pain Inventory
- Observation of pain-related behaviors such as guarded movement, facial grimacing, and protective posturing.

Scars:

- Burn Scar Index (Vancouver Scar Scale)
- Patient and Observer Scar Assessment Scale

INTERVENTION

EMERGENT PHASE:

- **Establish a splinting and positioning program** to prevent early contracture formation and reduce edema at first visit (see preventive/antideformity positioning in subsequent section).
- All joints with **a superficial partial-thickness burn or worse should be splinted**.
- **Provide psychological support.**

PLACE OF THERMAL INJURY & TYPICAL CONTRACTURE	PREVENTIVE/ANTIDEFORMITY POSITIONING: TECHNIQUE AND IMPLEMENTS
Anterior neck: Flexion	Neutral/slight extension: Extension splint or collar, remove pillows
Anterior shoulder: Adduction	120° Abduction with slight external rotation: Positioning wedges, airplane splint, arm boards, clavicle straps
Anterior elbow: Flexion	Elbow extension: Positioning wedges, conformer, or dynamic splint with 5°–10° flexion
Dorsal wrist: Extension	Neutral to 20° extension: Wrist splint
Volar wrist: Flexion	5–10° flexion: Wrist cockup splint

CONDITIONS

PLACE OF THERMAL INJURY & TYPICAL CONTRACTURE	PREVENTIVE/ANTIDEFORMITY POSITIONING: TECHNIQUE AND IMPLEMENTS
Dorsal hand: Claw hand deformity	Metacarpophalangeal (MCP) joints 70–90°, interphalangeal (IP) joints in full extension, thumb in opposition: Functional hand splint
Volar hand: Cupping of hand	MCP joints slightly hyperextended: Palm extension splint
Hip anterior: Flexion	Prone positioning, trochanter rolls, wedges, knee immobilizers
Knee: Flexion	Positioning in knee extension: Knee conformer, dynamic splints
Ankle: Plantar flexion	Ankle positioned in 90°: Splint, ankle foot orthosis (AFO), cast or foot board

Data from Pendleton, H., & Schultz-Krohn, W. (2017). *Pedretti's Occupational Therapy: Practice Skills for Physical Dysfunction (Occupational Therapy Skills for Physical Dysfunction (Pedretti)).* 8th ed. St. Louis, Missouri: Mosby.

ACUTE/SURGICAL PHASE:

- If skin grafting occurs, OT must **fabricate splints** to immobilize the area in antideformity positions (see preventive/antideformity positioning above).
- **Exercise program** should begin with passive range of motion (PROM) and progress through active range of motion (AROM) and therapeutic activity as appropriate.

Occupation-based intervention/ADL retraining:

- If possible, the patient should be encouraged to sit on the edge of bed to engage in feeding and basic self-care such as hygiene and grooming or upper body dressing. However, depending on the extent of the injury, s/he may be limited due to a complex medical status, in which case the focus of care should be to preserve range of motion and strength through positioning, splinting, and exercise.

REHABILITATIVE PHASE:

- **Activities of daily living/instrumental activities of daily living (ADLs/IADLs):** The goal is to return patient to

prior level of function at this stage. Use of adaptive equipment or compensatory techniques can be implemented if patient has difficulty with the activity.

- **Sensation**: It is common for areas to develop increased sensitivity. **Desensitization** is a process by which the therapist exposes the skin to soft textures (e.g., cotton balls or silk), slowly increasing exposure time and roughness of material (e.g., towel, wool). Gentle massage and vibration may also be used with caution.

- **Scar management:** After sufficient healing, the patient should be trained in **scar massage**; using lotion, moving fingertips in a circular motion with deep pressure, to be performed several times per day. **Pressure dressings** and garments should be worn starting at only a few hours per day until tolerance can be developed for 24-h wear. These may include pressure gloves, Coban, Tubigrip, or elastic bandages. Wraps are applied in spiral fashion distal to proximal and overlapping. Patients should also be instructed in **skin hygiene**; moisturizing daily, and using at least 30 sun protection factor (SPF) if exposed to sun.

- **Establish and train in a stretching program** (in addition to ROM program) throughout the scar maturation phase. This should first be performed by the OT, then monitored as the patient begins to takes over the program.

Occupation-based intervention/ADL retraining examples:

- The patient is engaged in a laundry-folding activity incorporating principles of desensitization of the residual limb. Prior to folding each garment, the patient is tasked with exposing the affected area to the different fabrics and textures as tolerated.

PROVIDING CLIENT-CENTERED CARE:

- Education and training are highly important regarding conditions or injuries in which the patient must take an active role in managing, as is the case with burns. In addition to retraining in areas of ADL/IADL the OT should encourage active participation in a splinting/ROM program, desensitization, and scar management.

Cardiovascular Disease

CARDIOCASCULAR DISEASE/HEART DISEASE

A variety of conditions affecting the heart and/or blood vessels are grouped together to comprise cardiovascular disease (CVD). It is estimated that 80% of CVD is preventable; however, it is the leading cause of death in the United States and globally (*CDC Prevention Programs*, 2018). The most important risk factors are modifiable lifestyle choices including poor diet, lack of physical activity, tobacco use, and alcohol consumption (*Cardiovascular diseases*, 2019). The patient's capacity to engage in activities of daily living (ADLs) and other meaningful activities is typically reduced in the setting of CVD. Accordingly, the patient should be educated in healthy lifestyle changes to prevent or manage the disease and ways to make such changes sustainable for long-term compliance.

CONDITION	
HEART DISEASE	LIFESTYLE MODIFICATIONS
AN UMBRELLA TERM FOR A RANGE OF CONDITIONS:	
• Coronary artery disease (CAD)	
1. A build-up of cholesterol and other fatty substances occurs in the walls of the arteries that supply the heart with blood.	• Weight loss/maintain healthy body mass index (BMI)
2. Deposits then turn to plaque, narrowing and hardening the artery (known as atherosclerosis).	• Exercise • Reduce stress • Heart-healthy diet • Manage blood pressure and cholesterol • Manage diabetes

HEART DISEASE	LIFESTYLE MODIFICATIONS
• **Heart rhythm abnormalities** Atrial fibrillation (A-fib) is the most common type of arrhythmia. 1. Abnormal electrical firing causes the four chambers of the heart to beat erratically. 2. The disorganized pumping causes a stagnation of blood flow in the atria causing clots to form. 3. Clots can travel to the cerebral arteries causing blockage/ischemia. • Congestive heart failure (CHF) 1. Occurs when conditions such as hypertension (HTN), CAD, myocardial infarction (MI), A-fib, etc. weaken the heart to the extent that it can no longer pump enough blood to meet the body's metabolic needs. 2. To compensate, the heart beats faster and the myocardium (heart muscle) thickens in order to pump more forcefully, leading to an enlarged heart. 3. Stroke may occur due to elevated blood pressure and increased incidence of blood clots. • **Heart attack/MI** 1. A build-up of cholesterol and other fatty substances collect in the walls of the arteries that supply the heart with blood. 2. Deposits then turn to plaque, narrowing and hardening the artery causing atherosclerosis. 3. A plaque can then rupture, form a clot, which occludes the artery, and consequently blocks blood flow to the heart, causing infarction.	• Limit sodium • Avoid alcohol • Smoking cessation

CONDITIONS

HYPERTENSION/HTN	LIFESTYLE MODIFICATIONS
1. High blood pressure causes damage to the arterial walls. 2. Fatty deposits begin to form in the microtears of the damaged walls. 3. Deposits then turn to plaque, narrowing and hardening the artery causing atherosclerosis.	• Weight loss/maintain healthy BMI • Exercise • Reduce stress • Dietary Approaches to Stop Hypertension (DASH) diet • Limit sodium • Smoking cessation • Lower cholesterol • Avoid alcohol

DIABETES MELLITUS (DM II)	LIFESTYLE MODIFICATIONS
1. A chronic metabollic disorder characterized by high blood glucose levels caused by insulin resistance and reduced insulin production. 2. The excess glucose damages the inner walls of the blood vessels including those of the heart. 3. Comorbid conditions associated with DM II also increase the risk of developing CVD. These include hypertension, high low-density lipoprotein (LDL), and high triglycerides.	• Diabetic diet • Exercise to increase insulin sensitivity • Weight loss/maintain healthy BMI • Smoking cessation

HIGH LDL	LIFESTYLE MODIFICATIONS
1. A build-up of cholesterol and other fatty substances collect in the walls of the arteries that supply the heart with blood. 2. Deposits then turn to plaque, narrowing and hardening the artery causing atherosclerosis.	• Weight loss/maintain healthy BMI • Exercise • Heart-healthy diet • Smoking cessation

ALCOHOL	LIFESTYLE MODIFICATIONS
• Causes hypertension. • Provokes episodes of A-fib. • Increases risk of developing DM II. • Prevents the coagulation function of the liver which can lead to hemorrhagic stroke.	• Community support programs/Alcoholics Anonymous (AA) • Counseling

SMOKING	LIFESTYLE MODIFICATIONS
• Increases blood pressure causing hypertension. • Increases the build-up of plaque, primarily in the carotid (neck) arteries. • Makes blood more likely to clot.	• Smoking cessation programs

OBESITY	LIFESTYLE MODIFICATIONS
Obesity, especially abdominal fat, is a high-risk factor for developing: • Cardiovascular disease. • High blood pressure causing hypertension. • Insulin resistance leading to diabetes. • Sleep apnea.	• Exercise • Mediterranean diet • Limit portion size • Track food intake • Avoid alcohol

SEDENTARY LIFESTYLE	LIFESTYLE MODIFICATIONS
A sedentary lifestyle is a high-risk factor for developing: • Excess body fat. • Blood clots. • High blood pressure. • High LDL.	• Home exercise program • Resources for community programs and recreational centers

Carlsson et al. (2013).

CONDITIONS

ASSESSMENT

Endurance:

- 6 Minute Walk Test (6MWT)

Functional ability & mobility:

- Modified Barthel Index (MBI)
- Canadian Occupational Performance Measure (COPM)
- Timed Up and Go (TUG)

Perceived exertion:

- Borg Rating of Perceived Exertion (RPE) Scale

Borg RPE Scale®

Use this scale to tell how strenuous and tiring the work feels to you. The exertion is mainly felt as fatigue in your muscles and as breathlessness or possibly aches. When the exercise is hard it also becomes difficult to talk. It is your own feeling of exertion that is important. Don't underestimate it, but don't overestimate it either. For common exercise, such as cycling, running or walking, 11-15 is a good level. For strength and high-intensity interval training (HIIT), 15-19 is good. If you are sick follow your doctor's advice. Look at the scale and the descriptions and then choose a number. Use whatever numbers you want, even numbers between the descriptions.

6	**No exertion at all**	No muscle fatigue, breathlessness or difficulty in breathing.
7	**Extremely light**	Very, very light.
8		
9	**Very light**	Like walking slowly for a short while. Very easy to talk.
10		
11	**Light**	Like a light exercise at your own pace.
12	**Moderate**	
13	**Somewhat hard**	Fairly strenuous and breathless. Not so easy to talk.
14		
15	**Hard**	Heavy and strenuous. An upper limit for fitness training, as when running or walking fast.
16		
17	**Very hard**	Very strenuous. You are very tired and breathless. Very difficult to talk.
18		
19	**Extremely hard**	The most strenuous effort you have ever experienced.
20	**Maximal exertion**	Maximal heaviness.

Borg RPE Scale®
Ratings (R) of Perceived (P) Exertion (E).
© Gunnar Borg, 1970, 1998, 2017
English

The Borg RPE Scale (R) ([C] Gunnar Borg, 1970, 1998, 2017). Scale printed with permission.

- The Borg Scale ranges from 6 to 20 as it is designed to provide the clinician with an estimate of the patient's **heart rate during activity**. This can be calculated by taking the patient's RPE number and multiplying it by 10. For example, if a patient rates her exertion as a '12' it should in theory correlate with a heart rate of about 120 (12 $\times$ 10 = 120).

INTERVENTION

- Educate in applicable **lifestyle modifications** (see previous section).
- **Early mobilization** in acute care/intensive care unit (ICU).
- Create a **home exercise program** that the patient can complete independently, outside of therapy.
- Instruct in techniques to **reduce edema**: Raise the affected limb higher than level of the heart, movement/pumping the extremity, use of compression garments such as a sleeve or stocking, and retrograde massage.
- Recommend and educate in use of **adaptive equipment** (AE) and **durable medical equipment** (DME) (see Additional Intervention: Adaptive Equipment).
- Instruct in **task modification and energy conservation** as they relate to activities of daily living/instrumental activities of daily living (ADLs/IADLs), including appropriate **breathing patterns** (see Education: Energy Conservation Techniques).
- Facilitate therapeutic activity to improve **functional activity tolerance**.
- Train in **stress management**: Relaxation techniques, deep breathing, and sleep hygiene (Shoemaker et al. (2020)).

Occupation-based intervention/ADL retraining examples:

- The occupational therapist (OT) collaborates with the patient to create a grocery list of heart-healthy foods and facilitates a meal preparation session using a recipe that is compliant with a heart-healthy diet.
- The OT educates the patient in energy conservation techniques and incorporates these principles into a showering task including use of shower chair, pursed-lip breathing, pacing, and tripod position (sits leaned forward supporting upper body weight through elbows which rest on the knees).

CONDITIONS

PROVIDING CLIENT-CENTERED CARE:

- In order to effect lasting lifestyle changes it is imperative to incorporate the patient's preferences in the areas of diet and activity. Healthy lifestyle changes can be difficult to sustain, thus capitalizing on choices that the patient identifies as appealing can help facilitate long term compliance.

19

Cerebral Vascular Accident/Stroke

CEREBRAL VASCULAR ACCIDENT

A cerebral vascular accident (CVA), also known as a stroke, occurs when either a blockage (ischemic stroke) or a brain bleed (hemorrhagic stroke) causes part of the brain to lose oxygen resulting in local death of tissue.

BE FAST stroke signs:

B—Balance. Is the person suddenly having trouble with balance or coordination?

E—Eyes. Is the person experiencing suddenly blurred or double vision or a sudden loss of vision in one or both eyes without pain?

F—Face Drooping. Does one side of the face droop or is it numb? Ask the person to smile. Is the person's smile uneven?

A—Arm Weakness. Is one arm weak or numb? Ask the person to raise both arms. Does one arm drift downward?

S—Speech Difficulty. Is speech slurred?

T—Time to call 911

Data from Fletcher, M. (n.d.). *Know the Signs of Stroke—BE FAST*. Duke Health. Retrieved October 22, 2021, from https://www.dukehealth.org/blog/know-signs-of-stroke-be-fast

CONDITIONS

ISCHEMIC	**Inadequate blood supply to an area of the brain due to partial or complete obstruction of an artery. Approximately 80% of all strokes are ischemic. Types of ischemic strokes are listed below.**
THROMBOTIC	A thrombosis (blood clot in the circulatory system) forms at the site of injury inside the arterial wall, blocking blood flow, causing infarction (death of tissue). As atherosclerotic plaques are interpreted as an injury by the body, thrombi generally form where the blood vessels are already narrowed.
EMBOLIC	A thrombosis becomes an embolus once it leaves the site where it developed and travels with blood flow. The term *embolus* also refers to other debris in the blood stream including pieces of plaque. Stroke occurs when the embolus becomes lodged, causing infarction.
TRANSIENT ISCHEMIC ATTACK/TIA	Also called a "mini" or "warning" stroke. A short-term blockage without infarction that typically resolves without intervention.
LACUNAR	A type of thrombotic stroke that occurs when a small artery serving the subcortical areas of the brain (basal ganglia, thalamus, internal capsule or pons) becomes occluded causing infarction.
HEMORRHAGIC	**A brain bleed that occurs in or around the brain when a weakened blood vessel ruptures. Types of hemorrhagic strokes are listed below.**
INTRACEREBRAL	A bleed into the brain tissue caused by a ruptured vessel, also known as an intracranial hemorrhage.
SUBARACHNOID	A bleed that occurs between the subarachnoid and pia mater meninges in the cerebrospinal fluid-filled space.
ANEURYSM	The ballooning of a weakened artery causing a stroke when ruptured, typically occurring in the circle of Willis.

LEFT BRAIN DAMAGE	RIGHT BRAIN DAMAGE
Right side motor and sensory loss	Left side motor and sensory loss
Right visual field cut	Left visual field cut
Expressive aphasia (Broca's area)	Left-sided neglect
Receptive aphasia (Wernicke's area)	Left spatial-perceptual deficits
Impaired right/left discrimination	Impulsive/impaired safety awareness
Insight into deficits, deliberate and cautious	Anosognosia (lack of insight into deficits)
Depression/anxiety	Impaired judgement
Impaired analytical thinking	Decreased attention span

Common underlying impairments caused by stroke that affect ability to safely and effectively perform activities of daily living/instrumental activities of daily living (ADLs/IADLs):

- Hyper/hypotonicity, limited range of motion, shoulder subluxation, limited trunk control leading to poor sitting and standing balance, thoracic kyphosis, shortened lateral trunk muscles, inability to bear weight through upper or lower extremities due to weakness or asymmetrical weight bearing, downward rotation of affected scapula, internal rotation of the affected humerus, high tone/contracture of affected biceps, supination of affected forearm with flexion of wrist and fingers.

Common ineffective movement strategies caused by stroke that affect ability to safely perform ADLs/IADLs:

- Inability to perform sit to stand or other functional transfers; inability to use proper hip, ankle, and stepping strategies to engage in dynamic movement; inability to bear weight equally through lower extremities decreasing stability of base of support (BOS); inability to use affected upper extremity to engage in ADLs; and development of abnormal, compensatory movement patterns.

CONDITIONS

ASSESSMENT

Basic:

- Range of motion (ROM)
- Manual muscle testing (MMT)
- Sensation
  - Semmes-Weinstein Monofilament Test
- Proprioception
- Tone
- Edema

Functional ability & mobility:

- Modified Barthel Index (MBI)
- Functional Independence measure (FIM)
- Lawton IADL Scale
- Performance Assessment of Self Care Skills (PASS)
- Timed Up and Go Test (TUG)
- Five Times Sit to Stand

Hand strength and coordination:

- Pinch and Grip Strength (Dynamometer)
- Purdue Pegboard tests
- Nine-hole Peg Test
- Chedoke Arm and Hand Activity Inventory
- Motor Evaluation Scale for Upper Extremity in Stroke Patients (MESUPES)

Balance/fall risk:

- Berg Balance Scale (BBS)
- Tinetti Balance and Gait Assessment
- Modified Clinical Test of Sensory Interaction in Balance (CTSIB-M)

Postural control:

- Postural Assessment Scale for Stroke (PASS)

Spasticity:

- Modified Ashworth Scale

Cognitive function:
- Clock Drawing Test
- Executive Function Performance Test (EFPT)
- Mini Mental State Examination (MMSE)
- Montreal Cognitive Assessment (MoCA)

Neurobehavioral/cognitive perceptual:
- Arnadottir Occupational Therapy Neurobehavioral Evaluation (A-ONE)

Visual function:
- Homonymous hemianopsia
  - Visual Field Test
- Unilateral neglect
  - Line bisection test
  - Cancellation test
  - Behavioral Inattention Test (BIT)
- Visual screening
  - See Conditions: Low Vision: Visual Screening

Ability to live independently:
- Kohlman Evaluation of Living Skills (KELS)
- Allen Cognitive Level Screen (ACLS)

Pain:
- Verbal Rating Scale
- 0–10 Numeric Pain Intensity Scale
- Wong Baker Faces Scale
- The Brief Pain Inventory
- Observation of pain-related behaviors such as guarded movement, facial grimacing, and protective posturing.

Depression:
- The Geriatric Depression Scale (GDS)
- Beck Depression Inventory (BDI)

Quality of life:
- Stroke-Specific Quality of Life (SS-QOL)

Comprehensive:

• Stroke Impact Scale

INTERVENTION

REMEDIAL TECHNIQUES

Abnormal tone:

• Traditional sensorimotor facilitatory techniques:

  • Heavy joint compression/approximation, tapping, quick stretch, brushing, cryotherapy, therapeutic vibration, e-stim.

• Traditional sensorimotor inhibitory techniques:

  • Neutral warmth, light joint compression/ approximation, slow stroking, deep pressure, prolonged stretch, slow rolling, and slow rocking.

Neuromuscular reeducation:

• Proprioceptive Neuromuscular Facilitation (PNF):

  • Promotes functional movement patterns through inhibition, facilitation, relaxing, and strengthening muscle groups, utilizing concentric, eccentric, and isometric contractions.

  • Technique examples: Hold-relax, contract-relax, quick stretch, rhythmic initiation, rhythmic stabilization, slow reversal hold, alternating isometrics, isotonic stabilizing reversals, and alternating holds. See Additional Intervention: PNF Patterns for upper extremity D1/D2 flexion and extension patterns.

• Neuro-developmental Treatment (NDT):

  • Remediation of ineffective movement strategies through the facilitation of functional activities that are designed to reduce underlying impairments.

• Upper extremity weight-bearing activities:

  • Facilitation of weight-bearing activities to improve proprioception, normalize tone, and improve strength.

• Constrained-induced movement therapy (CIMT):

  • Inhibiting use of the unaffected extremity in order to promote use of the affected side.

Soft tissue shortening/spasticity:

- Low-load prolonged stretch, passive range of motion (only move shoulder past 90° flexion and abduction if there is upward rotation of scapula and external rotation of the humerus), splinting program, soft tissue mobilization, bed positioning, and encouraging frequent movement including active-assistive range of motion.

Weakness:

- Establish and train in a home exercise program (HEP) to be performed throughout the week in addition to therapy.

Edema:

- Elevation above the level of the heart, compression garments, retrograde massage, pumping of the extremity, contrast baths, and positioning to prevent the extremity from hanging down for long periods. Refer to Conditions: Hand Injury and Impairment: Edema Control for treatment of edematous hand.

COMPENSATORY TECHNIQUES:

ADL/IADL performance:

- Hemiplegic techniques, task modification.
- Adaptive equipment recommendations (see Additional Intervention: Adaptive Equipment).

Changes in cognition:

- See Additional Intervention: ADL retraining techniques

Fall prevention:

- See Education: Fall Prevention

Fatigue:

- See Education: Energy conservation techniques

Low vision:

- See Conditions: Low Vision

Neglect:

- Visual scanning
  - **Lighthouse technique**: An organized search pattern in which patient turns head fully scanning from left to right with conscious attention to detail.

- **Anchoring (in environment):** Bright colored tape or other attention-grabbing objects placed on the affected side.
- **Anchoring (on paper):** A mark such as a line or a number placed at the beginning or end of a sentence to indicate the starting and/or ending place.
- **Letter cancellation:** Worksheets that facilitate scanning through the search of a particular letter or symbol among an array of characters.

- ADLs and other activities can be **performed in front of a mirror** to bring attention to the affected side.
- Caregiver training to approach and **talk to the patient on the affected side.**
- **Eye patching** and **prism glasses.**

Return to residence:

- **Home safety evaluation** with recommendations (see Assessment: Home Safety Eval/Checklist).
- Address **community mobility** and provide resources.
- Determine amount of assistance needed for ADLs/IADLs and **provide caregiver training** or community resources for obtaining caregiver.

Example of treatment progression:

Program should be flexible, integrated, and address multiple deficits concurrently. Meaningful activity based on hobbies and roles should be incorporated throughout treatment sessions.

- **Positioning** in bed to prevent decubitus ulcers (see Conditions: Pressure Ulcers).
- **Dysphagia intervention** (see Conditions: Dysphagia).
- Instruct in **management of the hemiparetic upper extremity** to prevent subluxation, soft tissue contractures, and pain.
- **Facilitatory and inhibitory techniques** (see previous section) to normalize muscle tone.
- Restore **scapulohumeral rhythm** through scapular mobilization.

- Ensure **scapulothoracic (proximal) stability** prior to distal mobility.
- Establish ability to **sit unsupported** while maintaining trunk in midline with erect spine and neutral pelvis or slight anterior pelvic tilt.
- Facilitate participation in **seated upper body ADLs**.
- Introduce **seated weight-shifting activities** that promote bilateral integration, crossing midline, and leaning/reaching outside BOS.
- Facilitate intervention to **increase/normalize somatosensory perception.**
- Engage patient in **fine motor tasks** incorporating hobbies and interests.
- Instruct in **hemiplegic ADL techniques**.
- Introduce **adaptive equipment** for temporary or permanent use as appropriate.
- Facilitate **PNF patterns** to restore normal movement (see Additional Intervention: PNF Patterns).
- Facilitate participation in **lower body ADLs**.
- Train in preparatory elements for **safe static and dynamic standing** including equal weight bearing through bilateral lower extremities, proper postural alignment, and adjustment/control.
- Educate in **transfer sequence** including sit <> stand and functional transfers to various surfaces.
- Design dynamic ipsilateral **reaching activities** to promote task-specific weight-shifting abilities.
- Engage the patient in activities to **remediate balance and vestibular dysfunction** and train in compensatory techniques.
- Train in **higher-level IADLs** such as cleaning and cooking using multiple postural adjustments and balance strategies as well as adaptive equipment to safely complete tasks.
- Provide strength training and functional activities designed to **build endurance**. (O'Sullivan et al. (2019).)

CONDITIONS

Occupation-based intervention/ADL retraining example:

The patient is instructed in toileting using a slide board to transfer from wheelchair to bedside commode and back. The occupational therapist (OT) first demonstrates and then guides patient through the activity. Two-step cues are given first to line the wheelchair up with a 45° angle to the bedside commode (which is placed so the patient is transferring toward the unaffected/stronger side) and then to remove footrest. Next the patient is instructed to pull up the arm of the wheelchair and drop the arm of the commode, with the OT providing assist throughout the process. The OT cues the patient to lean away and lift her leg in order to facilitate placement of the slide board. The OT then provides mod assistance to safely slide patient to bedside commode. The patient is physically cued to assist by bearing weight through her upper extremities while leaning toward the commode. Instruction is given to weight shift side to side in order to bring pants down over hips. The OT assists with perineal care and with bringing pants up over hips while patient leans side to side. The wheelchair is then brought to the other side so that the patient can transfer off of bedside commode onto the wheelchair toward the unaffected side. Once the patient has gained more postural stability and strength, the OT will guide the patient through transfering toward both the affected and unaffected sides.

OTHER CONSIDERATIONS

- **Early mobilization** is highly important. As soon as the patient is stable, s/he should be encouraged to participate in self-care activities.

- **Remedial techniques should be the primary focus** in the beginning of treatment, in order to take advantage of neuroplasticity; a patient will make the greatest gains in the first 3 to 6 months poststroke. Once patient begins to plateau, compensatory strategies can then be introduced. Similarly, adaptive equipment should only be utilized for irremediable impairments.

- **Discharge planning** should begin at start of care.

- Discuss **driver safety concerns** with patient and family due to any changes in vision, cognition, or motor skills and provide information regarding alternative options for transportation.

- Studies have found that nearly 30% of stroke survivors develop depression due to both biochemical and psychosocial changes (Towfighi et al., 2016). OT can **perform a basic depression screen** and report findings to referring MD.

PROVIDING CLIENT-CENTERED CARE:

- Collaborating with family can be highly beneficial if the patient's ability to communicate has been compromised. Family members can help to provide the OT with information regarding meaningful occupations and can assist with prioritizing needs on the patient's behalf. Family members can also be trained in providing assistance and carrying out protocols to help prepare for the transition home. It is important to note, however, that any information shared must be done so in a manner consistent with HIPAA guidelines to ensure the confidentiality and privacy of the patient's protected health information.

20

Dysphagia

Dysphagia is the dysfunction of any stage of swallow or the inability to swallow. It is often treated by the speech-language pathologist (SLP); however, in some facilities, it is treated primarily by the OT. In addition to deglutition, a multitude of performance skills are required to eat and drink safely and effectively including head and trunk control, upper extremity movement, oral control, and muscle tone with intact cognition, sensation, and perception. Refer to Analysis of Occupational Performance: Feeding and Deglutition for normal function.

INTERNATIONAL DYSPHAGIA DIET STANDARDIZATION INITIATIVE

Liquids

Level 0: Thin

- Fast flow such as water, tea, coffee, soda.

Level 1: Slightly thick

- Requires slightly more effort to drink than thin liquids, flows through a straw.

Level 2: Mildly thick/nectar thick

- Flows quickly from a spoon but slower than thin drinks.

Level 3: Moderately thick/honey thick

- Difficult to drink through a straw. Smooth texture with no lumps or fibers.

Level 4: Extremely thick/pudding thick

- Needs to be eaten with a spoon, cannot drink with straw.

Solids

Level 4: Puree

- Overlaps with liquid level 4. Pureed, cohesive, pudding-like foods that do not require formation of bolus or ability to chew.
  - Pudding, hummus, pureed fruits/vegetables, pureed meat.

Level 5: Minced and moist

- Foods that easily form into a bolus: moist, mashed, soft-textured, or finely minced. Minimal ability to chew is required.
  - Scrambled eggs, well-cooked vegetables, mashed potatoes. Meat, fish, or fruit that are finely minced.

Level 6: Soft and bite-sized

- Soft, tender, and moist foods that require more chewing.
  - Cooked/tender meat, stew, curry, cereal, steamed or boiled vegetables.

Level 7: Easy to chew/regular diet

- All foods allowed.

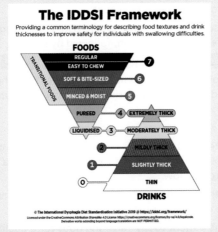

Data from The International Dysphagia Diet Standardisation Initiative 2019@ https://iddsi.org/framework/ Licensed under the CreativeCommons Attribution Sharealike 4.0 License. https://creativecommons.org/licenses/by-sa/4.0/legalcode.

ASSESSMENT

PREFEEDING ASSESSMENT:

- **Head and trunk control:**
  - Assess ability to maintain midline, tuck chin, and move head smoothly with sufficient range of motion (ROM).
- **Inner and outer oral status:**
  - Assess mobility of cheeks, jaw, lips, and tongue. Check for any bleeding or inflammation of gums.
  - Assess sensation of face and lips with cotton swab and ability to discern hot from cold using vials of different temperatures touched to lips or tongue.
  - Check for any primitive oral reflexes including suck-swallow, tongue thrust, or bite reflex.
- **Ability to protect airway:**
  - **Assess for intact palatal reflex:** Have patient say "ah" while increasing in pitch. Watch for elevation of uvula and contraction of faucial arches.
  - **Assess for elevation of the larynx:** Palpate the larynx and ask the patient to swallow. Feel for quick and smooth upward movement.
  - **Assess for productive cough:** Listen for strength and effectiveness of cough, followed by swallow.

FEEDING ASSESSMENT:

If the above functions are intact, the patient can then be presented with foods of various pureed/soft textures for trial.

- Place ½ teaspoon of food on patient's tongue.
- Palpate hyoid notch and larynx, feel for quality of swallow, and determine if the patient requires a second or third swallow.
- Note the transit time from initiating tongue movement to the end of the swallow process.
- Ask the patient to say "ah" and note voice quality and any pocketing.

FACTORS THAT INCREASE LIKELIHOOD OF ASPIRATION:

Oral phase impairments:

- Difficulty forming seal with mouth, managing secretions, or chewing solid foods. Inability to form bolus or move it to back of mouth, pocketing.

Pharyngeal phase impairments:

- If closure of the larynx does not occur, food, liquid, and other particulates can enter the lungs causing injury and infection known as aspiration pneumonia. Symptoms during mealtime include
  - Change in voice quality
  - Coughing
  - Choking

Esophageal phase impairments:

- Regurgitation, heartburn, burping, vomiting.

FLUID ASSESSMENT:

- Begin trial with level 3 (honey-thick) fluid, then progress through level 2 (nectar-thick), level 1 (flavored thin liquid), and finally level 0 (thin).
- The same sequence of the feeding assessment applies.
- If the patient has a wet, gargling sound in throat, s/he should be downgraded.

ADDITIONAL TESTING:

- A videofluoroscopy study (VSS), also known as a modified barium swallow (MBS) study, can be performed to determine if and why aspiration is occurring.

INTERVENTION

PREORAL AND ORAL STAGES:

- **Educate in proper positioning:** Seated on a firm surface, the patient's head and trunk should be in midline with chin slightly tucked. Hips are flexed to approximately 90° with an erect spine to prevent sacral sitting. Knees should be flexed to 90° and feet should rest comfortably on the floor.

CONDITIONS

- **Facilitate exercises** to promote strength, coordination, and increased ROM of oral structures.

- **Recommend appropriate adaptive equipment** (see Additional Intervention: Adaptive Equipment: Feeding).

- Place food on unimpaired side of mouth and tilt head toward same side.

PHARYNGEAL STAGE:

- **Facilitate tongue elevation** by gently pushing up underneath the patient's chin, at the base of the tongue.

- Alternate foods of **different temperatures**.

- **Infuse bolus** with lemon juice or other sour taste.

- **Instruct in compensatory techniques** including chin tuck, effortful swallow, neck rotation, supraglottic swallow, and the Mendelsohn maneuver.

- **Instruct in clearing throat** after each swallow or swallowing multiple times to ensure food has cleared.

ESOPHAGEAL STAGE:

- Therapists do not treat impairments at this stage of swallow.

Occupation-based intervention/activity of daily living (ADL) retraining example:

- A feeding and swallow assessment of a patient with a recent cerebral vascular accident (CVA) reveals poor positioning and dysfunction of the oral and pharyngeal stages of swallow. The occupational therapist (OT) repositions the patient to be in midline and corrects sacral sitting/posterior pelvic tilt by assisting the patient to bring her bottom to the back of the wheelchair. The OT first trains the patient in performing the Mendelsohn maneuver with saliva only. The patient is instructed to find the laryngeal prominence and feel how it elevates with swallowing. She is then instructed to attempt to keep it raised for 3 seconds during five swallows. Next, the OT trains in effortful swallow by cueing the patient to squeeze the muscles of the tongue and throat while swallowing a small spoonful of mashed potatoes.

The increased pressure generated by the throat and tongue helps to push and squeeze the bolus toward the esophagus. The OT cues the patient to place the mashed potatoes on the unimpaired side of her mouth and tilt her head toward the same side while also slightly tucking chin. After each swallow, she is instructed to clear her throat to prevent food particles from remaining.

OTHER CONSIDERATIONS

- The OT should **adhere to specific state and facility protocols** when entering diet texture/liquid consistency recommendations as orders.

- Supervision/assistance is recommended for **patients with poor attention** to feeding task, dementia, or motor impairments causing difficulty with self-feeding.

- **Gloves are mandatory** during assessments in order to be compliant with universal precautions.

- **Proper oral care** is essential in order to prevent aspiration of food particles and to decrease amount of bacteria and germs entering airway.

PROVIDING CLIENT-CENTERED CARE:

- During a dysphagia assessment/treatment session, food and drink choices may be limited by dietary restrictions and available menu items; however, the OT should still attempt to offer a few different options as able. Allowing the patient to make a decision based on personal preferences can help to foster a sense of agency and control over his or her care.

CONDITIONS

21

Fracture

FRACTURE

A fracture is a partial or complete break of a bone. The surgeon repairs the fracture site by first repositioning (reducing) bone fragments back into alignment. This is performed as either an open (operative) or closed (nonoperative) reduction. The bones can then be held together through internal fixation (known as open reduction internal fixation [ORIF]) with implants such as pins, plates, or screws. In the case of an external fixator, rods are placed into the bone, exiting through small incisions in the muscle and skin and attached to a stabilizing structure external to the body. Casting and splints may also be used. Occupational therapy (OT) intervention will vary greatly depending upon the manner in which the bone was fixed and the surgeon's treatment protocol.

ASSESSMENT

Ensure adherence to all precautions during assessments.

Basic:

- Range of motion (ROM)
- Manual muscle testing (MMT)
  - ROM and strength of affected joint to be assessed once permitted.

Functional ability & mobility:

- Modified Barthel Index (MBI)
- Functional Independence Measure (FIM)
- Lawton Instrumental Activities of Daily Living (IADL) Scale
- Timed Up and Go Test (TUG)

Balance & fall risk:

- Berg Balance Scale (BBS)

Pain:

- Verbal Rating Scale
- 0–10 Numeric Pain Intensity Scale
- Wong Baker Faces Scale
- Brief Pain Inventory

INTERVENTION

HUMERAL FRACTURE (NONOPERATIVE AND OPEN REDUCTION INTERNAL FIXATION [ORIF]):

- A **comprehensive shoulder protocol** is beyond the scope of this pocketbook but should be followed as set forth (or approved) by the referring surgeon for optimal healing.

- Although treatment programs may vary, the general guideline is to begin **Codman's pendulum exercises** by the second or third day post operatively, and progress through **partial passive range of motion** (PROM) and **isometric exercises** until week 6, at which point clinical union of the bone has likely occurred. If union is confirmed, the patient can begin **progressive exercises** for shoulder flexion, extension, abduction, and internal and external rotation.

- **Take caution** with Codman's exercises if upper extremity is edematous.

- Sling should be worn continuously for **3–6 weeks** unless performing ROM program, bathing, dressing, or carrying out hygiene and grooming tasks (ensure all movement occurs below the shoulder joint only).

- **No lifting, pushing, or pulling.**

- Instruct in completing transfers **without pushing up or lowering down using affected upper extremity.**

- Instruct in removal of sling for **active range of motion** (AROM) of **elbow, wrist, and hand** three to four times daily to prevent stiffness/contractures.

- Gentle, **nonresistive activities of daily living** (ADLs) should begin as soon as patient is cleared to do so. This might include **self-feeding** and **teeth brushing**, as long as they can be completed within the allowed ROM.

Occupation-based intervention/ADL retraining examples:

- The OT sets up a hygiene and grooming activity by removing the patient's sling and placing a tray table close to his body while seated at the edge of bed. The patient is able to access implements easily without having to reach (avoiding any movement of the shoulder joint). The OT educates the patient in shoulder precautions and provides verbal cues to ensure that only elbow, wrist, and hand movements occur throughout the activity. The patient is then guided through AROM below shoulder to prevent stiffness/contractures prior to replacing sling.

HAND/WRIST FRACTURE:

- **Distal radius fracture:** Train in **AROM** of **shoulder, elbow** (if not casted), and **fingers**, as well as **tendon gliding exercises** to prevent stiffness and reduce edema; to be completed every 2 h for 5–10 reps each, holding end position for a few seconds. If patient has external fixator, train in **pin site care**. After fixator or cast is removed, patient will likely be prescribed a volar wrist splint. **Request protocol** from surgeon for **forearm and wrist ROM**. Various **fine motor exercises** can gradually be added to treatment.

- **Hand or finger fracture:** Instruct in **edema control, AROM** of unaffected joints, and **pain control**. Guide patient through the **referring surgeon's specific protocol**, which will likely include a **short period of immobility** followed by **splinting, active movement**, and, once bony healing occurs, **resistive exercises**.

FEMUR FRACTURE (OPEN REDUCTION INTERNAL FIXATION [ORIF]/PINNING):

- Generally, patients are **non-weight-bearing** (NWB), toe-touch (TTWB), or partial weight-bearing (PWB given in terms of a percentage, such as 50% weight-bearing) for the first **6–8 weeks** and eventually progressed to weight-bearing as tolerated (WBAT).

- Instruct in completing **ADLs** while **maintaining weight-bearing restrictions**.

- For **partial weight-bearing status**, the patient should be trained in **utilizing a scale** during ADLs in order to become familiar with the allowed amount of pressure that can be placed through the extremity. For example, a 200-lb patient has a 25% partial weight-bearing restriction and therefore should not support more than 50 lb with the affected extremity. The scale can be used during functional tasks to ensure compliance throughout all standing activity.

- In order to adhere to weight-bearing restrictions with transfers, instruct in performing sit to stands by **placing the operated lower extremity out** from the chair and lifting body weight with unaffected lower extremity as well as pushing up on arm rests. When transitioning from stand to sit, the patient should also **bear weight through the unaffected extremities**, in this case by again extending operated extremity out in front and lowering down by placing weight through the upper extremities on the arm rests.

- **Train in use of adaptive equipment**, which may include long-handled reacher, dressing stick, sock-aid, long-handled shoehorn, foot funnel, shower chair, and raised toilet seat.

Occupation-based intervention/ADL retraining example:

- The patient is 2 weeks status post (s/p) ORIF with PWB status. The OT facilitates a lower body dressing activity by first instructing the patient in proper sequencing: In sitting, she is cued to thread the operated lower extremity through the pant leg first, followed by the unoperated side. The OT instructs her to extend the operated foot out in order to decrease the amount of weight that is supported through this extremity as she stands up. She is given verbal cues to stand by pushing up with the unoperated lower extremity and by using the arm rests as well, while watching a scale placed under the operated extremity for visual feedback. She then hikes her pants over her hips while continuing to watch the scale to ensure that she is maintaining her weight-bearing precaution throughout the activity.

CONDITIONS

OTHER CONSIDERATIONS

- The OT can **request a protocol from the surgeon** or submit a protocol for approval with the understanding that the patient's progression through the program will be based on his or her individual healing and recovery.

- The OT should **endorse ambulation device** as prescribed by physical therapy (PT) following hip and knee surgery.

PROVIDING CLIENT-CENTERED CARE:

- It is important to understand how an impairment affects daily occupations as well as other aspects of the patient's life that are less apparent. This could include roles or obligations, such as: Is the patient a caretaker for a loved one? Can he perform his required duties as an employee? How might the impairment affect his ability to obtain groceries or other necessities? By completing a thorough interview at time of evaluation the OT can construct a comprehensive plan of care, ensuring participation in all aspects of life.

22

Hand Injury and Impairment

HAND INJURY AND IMPAIRMENT

Referral to a certified hand therapist (CHT) may be indicated depending on the severity of the injury. CHTs generally practice in the outpatient setting, thus patients must typically wait until discharge from hospital, skilled nursing facility, or home health services to be treated by a CHT. This is due to Medicare guidelines that require discharge from inpatient and home health services prior to initiating outpatient visits. Some exceptions may apply.

ASSESSMENT

Basic:
- Range of motion (ROM)
- Manual muscle testing (MMT)
- Sensation
  - Semmes-Weinstein Monofilament Test
- Grip and pinch strength/dynamometer
- Prehensile patterns
- Edema

Dexterity/coordination:
- Nine-Hole Peg Test
- Jebsen Test of Hand Function
- Sollerman Hand Function Test

Pain:

- Verbal Rating Scale
- 0–10 Numeric Pain Intensity Scale
- Wong Baker Faces Scale
- The Brief Pain Inventory
- Observation of pain-related behaviors such as guarded movement, facial grimacing, and protective posturing.

INTERVENTION (GENERAL)

Activities to improve fine motor coordination:

- See Occupation/Activity-Based Treatment Ideas: Fine Motor Skills

Edema control:

- Elevation, compression, retrograde massage, active movement, contrast baths: alternating hand between cold and warm water for 1 min each for a total of 20 min, ending with cold water, and using a sponge for the patient to squeeze in each tub. Place tubs as high as possible to keep the hand elevated throughout the activity.

Tendon glides:

- The hand has two groups of flexor tendons: the flexor digitorum profundus and flexor digitorum superficialis, which are held together in a sheath. These tendons must function together and individually (known as differential gliding) within the sheath to produce coordinated and pain-free movements.

- Tendon glides are indicated for a broad array of conditions in which the flexor tendons have been injured. This list includes but is not limited to repetitive stress injuries, carpal tunnel syndrome, trauma from surgery, and includes conditions in which the patient is prone to developing adhesions such as with rheumatoid or osteoarthritis. The exercises in figure "Tendon Glides" facilitate maximal differential glide of all flexor tendons across all joints, promoting optimal hand function.

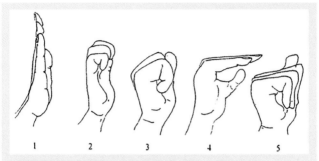

Tendon glides. (Adopted from Akalin, E., El, O., Peker, O., Senocak, O., Tamci, S., Gülbahar, S., et al. [2002]. Treatment of carpal tunnel syndrome with nerve and tendon gliding exercises. *American Journal of Physical Medicine & Rehabilitation, 81*[2], 108–113.)

Nerve glides:

- An injured or compressed nerve can become inflamed and entrapped in the surrounding soft tissue. The most common peripheral nerve entrapment syndrome is carpal tunnel syndrome, involving the medial nerve, followed by cubital tunnel syndrome, which involves the ulnar nerve (Cutts, 2007). Symptoms may include paresthesia, weakness, fine motor impairment, and sharp or shooting pain. See Assessment: Common Upper Extremity Conditions with Special Orthopedic Tests for evaluation of ulnar and median nerve entrapment.

- Nerve glides can help to restore normal sliding of the nerve and encourage pain-free movement. Median nerve glides are illustrated in figure "Median Nerve Glides" for conservative management of carpal tunnel syndrome.

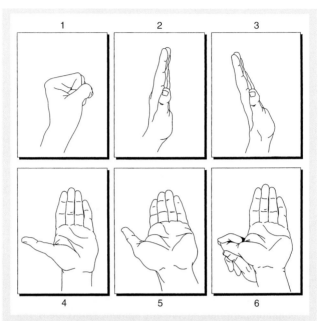

Median nerve glides. (Redrawn from Totten, P. A., & Hunter, J. M. [1991]. Therapeutic techniques to enhance nerve gliding in thoracic outlet syndrome and carpal tunnel syndrome. *Hand Clinics, 7*[3], 505–520. Mackin, E., Callahan, A. D., Skirven, T. M., et al. [Eds.]. [2002]. *Rehabilitation of the hand and upper extremity* [5th ed.]. St Louis: Mosby.)

INTERVENTION (SPECIFIC)

Carpal tunnel syndrome: Median nerve glides, tendon glides, wrist brace worn at night, thumb stretches to open carpal tunnel, and improvement in seated/standing postural alignment. Identify activities that strain the median nerve through wrist flexion/extension and modify tasks to avoid such motions.

Complex regional pain syndrome (CRPS): Warm, moist compress, gentle desensitization, transcutaneous electrical nerve stimulation (TENS), retrograde massage, active range of motion (AROM) of entire upper extremity, and contrast baths. Guide in stress-loading activities ("scrubbing and carrying"). Scapular mobilization can help to decrease shoulder pain and stiffness often associated with CRPS.

Cubital tunnel syndrome: Edema control, elbow pad splint, ulnar nerve glides. Avoid prolonged elbow flexion.

De Quervain tenosynovitis: Thumb spica splint, tendon glides, provide education in limiting repetitive thumb motions, recommend utensils with built-up handles. Avoid excessive ulnar and radial wrist deviation.

Extensor carpi ulnaris tendinitis: Ulnar gutter or wrist cockup splint.

Extensor pollicis longus tendinitis: Thumb spica splint, identify activities that provoke the tendon (repetitive thumb motions) in order to train in task modification.

Flexor carpi radialis tendinitis: Wrist cock-up splint in neutral.

Flexor carpi ulnaris tendinitis: Ulnar gutter splint. Educate in avoiding wrist flexion with ulnar deviation.

Flexor tenosynovitis (trigger finger): Metacarpophalangeal (MCP) extension stretches, massage, tendon glides, oval 8 splint. Surgical intervention may be indicated for release of A1 pulley.

Hand or finger fracture: See Conditions: Fracture

Low median nerve injury: A splint that positions the thumb in palmar abduction and slight opposition with digital MCP flexion and interphalangeal (IP) extension.

Low radial nerve injury: A dynamic splint that places wrist, MCPs, and thumb in slight extension to protect extensor tendons while healing.

Low ulnar nerve injury: A dynamic ulnar nerve splint that blocks hyperextension of MCPs of the small and ring fingers but still allows for full MCP flexion.

Osteoarthritis of hand: Recommendation of specific splint will depend on which joints are affected and the patient's lifestyle.

- Common orthoses include resting- and working-hand splints, carpometacarpal (CMC) stabilizing splints, and oval 8 or ring splints for finger joints.

CONDITIONS

- See Education: Joint Protection Principles.
- See Additional Intervention: Adaptive Equipment.
- Please refer to Chapter 25, p117 for specific hand exercises.
  - Skilled clinical judgment should be used to determine and prescribe specific exercises including number of repetitions.

Rheumatoid arthritis (RA): Forearm-based resting hand splints, joint protection techniques (see Education: Joint Protection Principles), adaptive equipment (see Additional Intervention: Adaptive Equipment). **RA of fingers:** Oval 8 splint for finger joint instability including Swan Neck or Boutonniere deformity.

Trigger finger: See flexor tenosynovitis above

Data from Trombly, C. A., Radomski, M. V., & Latham, C. A. T. (2002). *Occupational Therapy for Physical Dysfunction.* Lippincott Williams & Wilkins.

Occupation-based intervention/activity of daily living (ADL) retraining example:
- The patient, a computer engineer, seeks conservative treatment for carpal tunnel syndrome. Upon recommendation by the occupational therapist (OT), the patient has obtained a split-and-tented keyboard as well as a vertical mouse. These ergonomic tools allow the patient to maintain a more neutral wrist position as opposed to a traditional keyboard and mouse, which promote wrist extension, pronation, and ulnar deviation. While the patient sits at his workstation, the OT uses physical cues to improve postural alignment and recommends raising his monitor to eye level. The patient is then guided through a series of tendon and nerve glides as well as thumb stretches, which the OT recommends he perform three times throughout his workday.

PROVIDING CLIENT-CENTERED CARE:
- The majority of treatment protocols for hand and wrist injury or impairment require a short period of immobility, which is typically managed by splinting. The OT can

collaborate with the patient in order to create a wearing schedule that is aligned with her daily routine. For example, this would take into account self-care activities, range-of-motion (ROM) programs, and any other occupations that require removal of the splint. By tailoring the program to fit the patient's schedule, the OT is acknowledging that his daily routines, activities, and preferences are important and need to be considered, which will likely increase compliance and engagement as well.

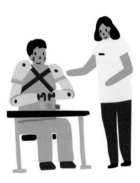

23

Low Vision

LOW VISION

Low vision refers to vision loss that cannot be corrected by usual means such as glasses, medical, or surgical intervention. Common diagnoses that may bring about low vision include macular degeneration, diabetic retinopathy, cataracts, glaucoma, and multiple sclerosis.

VISUAL SCREENING

Eye alignment:
- Hirschberg technique: A light is shined into the eyes, and if aligned, the corneal reflection will be in the same location on both eyes.

Visual fixation:
- Test the patient's ability to hold her gaze on a stationary object located approximately 2 feet from her eyes. The object should be held at midline, then held to the right and left sides. Normal findings: The patient should be able to hold her gaze for 10 s without eye or head movement.

Saccades:
- Hold two fingers approximately 1 foot apart from each other and 18 inches in front of the patient's eyes. Ask the patient to look at one target and then the next at random intervals for 30 s. Normal findings: Quick, accurate eye movements to each target without moving head or over/under shooting target.

Smooth pursuit:
- Use a finger or pen to slowly draw the letter "H" in the air approximately 18 inches from the patient's eyes. Ask the patient to track the pattern of the letter. Normal findings: The ability to direct gaze in all directions.

Convergence:

- A fixation target is placed 2 feet from the patient's eyes and is then moved slowly towards the patient's nose. Ask the patient to report when the target doubles. Normal findings: Patient should not see doubling of target outside of 6 inches from face.

Distal visual acuity:

- Assessed using Snellen chart. Patient stands 20 feet from the chart using eyewear, if prescribed. Each eye is tested separately and then together. Record the lowest line in which the patient can read more than half of the letters. Normal findings: 20/20; 20/30–20/60 is considered near-normal vision or mild vision loss.

Near visual acuity:

- Assessed using any type of document (e.g., handouts, newspaper, magazine, etc.). Paper is held 14–16 inches from eyes using eyewear, if prescribed. Point to six different letters, asking patient to identify each. Normal findings: Correctly identifies at least five out of six letters.

INTERVENTION

Lighting:

- Although each patient will have unique sensitivities to different types of lights, the general guidelines are as follows:
  - **Task lighting**: Light-emitting diode (LED) lighting in an adjustable, angled style lamp (to shine light on work surface rather than eyes) is best for specific tasks.
  - **General/ambient lighting:** Compact fluorescent lamp (CFL) bulbs are best for general lighting as they are known to reduce glare and eye strain.
  - Use of **lighted magnifying glass** if the above lighting is insufficient.

Contrast strategies:

- **Use of bright colors** for frequently used items such as a neon case for cellphone, brightly painted keys, red placemats, or **contrast tape** placed on the edge of the remote or call light. Contrast tape can also be used on the edge of stairs and on grab bars for safety.

Organization/clutter reduction:
- Establish a consistent routine with objects and implements **kept in specific places**.
- **Reduce clutter** on surfaces and **organize supplies** so that frequently used items can remain within reach.

Sensory substitution:
- **Use of other senses** as a compensatory measure. For example, feeling for tags on clothing, using auditory reading aids/books on tape, or a talking watch.
- **Bump dots** can be used on various surfaces including appliances, oven/stovetop, or medication bottles. (Muntges (n.d.))

Occupation-based intervention/activity of daily living (ADL) retraining examples:
- The occupational therapist (OT) first inquires regarding the sequence in which the patient completes hygiene and grooming tasks in the morning. In this instance, the patient prefers to wash her hands, put in her clean denture, brush her hair, and finally put on makeup. The OT instructs the patient or caregiver in lining up the appropriate implements from left to right on bathroom counter so that patient can access each item in preferred sequential order. On the other side of the counter, the OT places facewash and denture cup/brush, which can be easily accessed in order for the patient to be prepared for her nighttime hygiene and grooming routine. The OT also instructs in returning implements to their specific place for future use.
- Specific to home health patients: The OT assists with placing bump dots on washer and dryer to delineate different settings. The OT collaborates with patient to create a color system for organizing clothes in the closet. The patient then folds and puts laundry away based on the new system.

OTHER CONSIDERATIONS

- Many communities have **state- or county-funded programs** for people with low vision offering services and resources. The OT may assist the patient in making a referral.
- If the patient is somewhat tech savvy, **apps** such as Microsoft's Seeing AI or Be My Eyes may be helpful.
- Some companies, such as ScriptAbility, offer **talking prescription labels** for medications.

PROVIDING CLIENT-CENTERED CARE:

- OTs are highly skilled in determining how an impairment impacts function through observing and assessing performance. However, as is the case with any injury or impairment, it is crucial to approach the patient with an open mind and practice active listening, in order to gain a deeper understanding of their experience with the disability.

CONDITIONS

24

Multiple Sclerosis

MULTIPLE SCLEROSIS

Multiple sclerosis (MS) is a disorder of the central nervous system (CNS) characterized by autoimmune attacks on the myelin sheaths covering nerve cells, resulting in sclerotic plaques. These plaques (also referred to as lesions or scar tissue) cause a disruption in axonal communication and may lead to varying degrees of motor impairment, disturbed sensory perception, fatigue, visual changes, cognitive deficits, spasticity, bowel/bladder changes, ataxic gait, and pain (Moreno-Torres et al., 2019). The most common disease course is a relapsing- (at least 24 h of worsening symptoms) remitting (partial or complete recovery) pattern. Relapses are also known as attacks, flares, or exacerbations and typically last 1–3 weeks but can last longer than 6 months.

ASSESSMENT

Basic:

- Range of motion (ROM)
- Manual muscle testing (MMT)
- Sensation
  - Semmes-Weinstein Monofilament Test (SWMT)

Functional ability & mobility:

- Modified Barthel Index (MBI)
- Functional Independence Measure (FIM)
- Performance Assessment of Self-care Skills (PASS)
- Canadian Occupational Performance Measure (COPM)
- Lawton Instrumental Activity of Daily Living (IADL) Scale
- Timed Up and Go Test (TUG)

Balance & fall risk:
- The Berg Balance Scale (BBS)
- Tinetti Balance and Gait Assessment
- Modified Clinical Test of Sensory Interaction in Balance (CTSIB-M)

Fatigue:
- Modified Fatigue Impact Scale (MFIS)
- Fatigue Descriptive Scale (FDS)

Cognitive function:
- Brief International Cognitive Assessment for MS (BICAMS)
- Montreal Cognitive Assessment (MoCA)
- Symbol Digit Modalities Test (SDMT)
- MS Neuropsychological Screening Questionnaire (MSNQ)

Spasticity:
- Modified Ashworth Scale

Vision:
- See Conditions: Low Vision: Visual Screening

Pain:
- Verbal Rating Scale
- 0–10 Numeric Pain Intensity Scale
- Wong Baker Faces Scale
- Brief Pain Inventory
- Observation of pain-related behaviors such as guarded movement, facial grimacing, and protective posturing.

Depression:
- The Beck Depression Inventory (BDI)
- Chicago Multiscale Depression Inventory

Ability to live independently:
- Kohlman Evaluation of Living Skills (KELS)
- Allen Cognitive Level Screen (ACLS)

Quality of life:
- Multiple Sclerosis Quality of Life-54 (MSQOL-54)

INTERVENTION

Fatigue:

The following exercise recommendations are meant to serve as general guidelines only and should not take the place of skilled clinical judgment based on individual assessment findings.

- **Strengthening programs** have proven to be protective against fatigue in the MS population (Bahmani et al., 2019), though they require careful monitoring. Exercises may be performed against gravity only, with rubber tubing, or weights and should be in three sets of 3–5 reps per the National MS Society (*Exercise*, 2021).

- **Walking, yoga, leg cycling, and aquatic** exercises have been found to reduce various symptoms of MS including fatigue (Halabchi et al., 2017). Aerobic activity should last 15–20 min and should be completed four to five times per week according to the National MS Society guidelines (*Exercise*, 2021).

- Educate in **preventing elevated body temperature** as this exacerbates fatigue.

- **Avoid overexertion** (see Education: Energy Conservation Techniques).

- **Explore power options** for community mobility and in advanced cases, an appropriate seating system for activities of daily living (ADL)-related mobility in the home.

Spasticity:

- **Prolonged passive stretching**: Develop a stretching program holding each stretch for 30–60 s.

- **Active or passive range of motion (A/PROM):** For rigidity, stiffness, or contractures. Train patient and/or caregivers in a basic ROM program to be completed daily.

- **Timing:** If taking baclofen or any other antispasticity drug, try to time stretching or PROM program for 1 h after it is administered.

- **Use positioning:** Patient should lie prone for spastic hip and knee flexors and on their side for hip and knee extensor spasticity.
- **Splinting, casting, or bracing** can also be effective in reducing spasticity.

Adaptive equipment for ADL impairment:

- **Feeding:** Utensils with built-up handles, lightweight utensils, U-cuff.
- **Dressing**: Dressing stick, sock aid, long-handled shoehorn or foot funnel, button hook.
- **Bathing:** Shower chair/transfer bench, grab bars, long-handled sponge, modify bathtub to walk-in shower in order to accommodate rolling chair if indicated and feasible.
- **Hygiene and grooming:** Electric toothbrush, long-handled hairbrush.
- **Toileting:** Bidet, long-handled tissue aid, riser, bedside commode, grab bars.

Visual changes:

- Low vision assessment and intervention (see Conditions: Low Vision).

Pain:

- Pain assessment and intervention (see Conditions: Pain).

Dysphagia:

- Dysphagia (see Conditions: Dysphagia), Speech-Language Pathology (SLP) referral.

Occupation-based intervention/ADL retraining examples:

- The OT facilitates a therapy session focused on dishwashing, as the patient reports difficulty completing this task with complaints of fatigue and low back pain. He is given verbal cues to stand against the sink and bring each dish as close to his body as possible while maintaining good postural alignment to reduce leaning forward while scrubbing and rinsing (proper body mechanics). He is also instructed to open the cupboard door and rest one foot on the inside to take pressure off the lower back, alternating feet every few minutes (joint protection principle). The occupational therapist (OT) educates in energy conservation techniques including pacing, recommending he rest prior to feeling fatigued. The OT then demonstrates movement in accordance with intra-abdominal pressure, instructing the patient to inhale while reaching up and exhale when reaching down. The patient returns demonstration by inhaling while reaching to put dishes in cupboard and exhaling to reach down into dishwasher.

- A patient reports she is no longer able to ambulate to the bathroom at night due to lower extremity weakness. As a remedial approach, the OT works collaboratively with the patient to create a strengthening program including use of a resistance band and leg cycling in order to improve lower extremity strength, which is to be completed outside of therapy. OT checks in with physical therapy to prevent any duplication of services from occurring. As an immediate compensatory measure, the OT recommends use of bedside commode at night. The spouse is trained in facilitating a stand pivot transfer and in providing assistance with clothing management to ensure patient's safety.

OTHER CONSIDERATIONS

- **Depression** is a common symptom of MS (Persson et al., 2020). A basic depression screening can be administered by the OT. Results should be reported to the referring MD.

- **Sleep disturbances** are also common and can exacerbate fatigue (Al-Sharman et al., 2019). The OT can educate in sleep hygiene and should report any sleep issues to the referring MD.

- If a patient presents with **cognitive deficits**, a standardized assessment may be indicated. This is especially prudent if the patient lives alone, as his or her safety could be at risk.

PROVIDING CLIENT-CENTERED CARE:

- Occupational performance and mobility may vary greatly due to the relapsing-remitting nature of MS. It is important to determine functional levels during an exacerbation, which may not be captured during time of evaluation. In order to create an optimal treatment plan that considers variable performance in the setting of MS, the OT can administer the Modified Fatigue Impact Scale or conduct a thorough interview inquiring specifically about functional levels during a flare.

CONDITIONS

25

Osteoarthritis (OA/DJD)

OSTEOARTHRITIS (OA)/DEGENERATIVE JOINT DISEASE (DJD)

Osteoarthritis is characterized by a breakdown of articular cartilage, which reduces joint space and causes painful bone-on-bone contact. Reactive new bone formations known as osteophytes may occur, causing the joint to lose its regular shape. A patient will generally experience stiff and painful joints and present with limited range of motion (ROM), poor strength, and crepitus—a rubbing or popping sound caused by the abnormal cartilage surfaces.

ASSESSMENT

Basic:

- Range of motion (ROM)
- Manual muscle testing (MMT)

Functional ability and mobility:

- Modified Barthel Index (MBI)
- Canadian Occupational Performance Measure (COPM)
- Timed up and Go Test (TUG)

Balance & Fall Risk:

- Berg Balance Scale (BBS)
- Tinetti Balance and Gait Assessment

Pain:

- Verbal Rating Scale
- 0–10 Numeric Pain Intensity Scale
- Wong Baker Faces Scale
- The Brief Pain Inventory

Comprehensive:

- Short-form Arthritis Impact Measurement Scales 2 (AIMS2-SF)

INTERVENTION

Decrease pain:

- **Bracing or splinting** to provide support for painful and unstable joints. Common splints include resting-, working-, and carpometacarpal joint (CMC)-stabilizing splints, while oval 8 or ring splints can be used for joints of fingers.

- Use of **therapeutic modalities:**

  - Superficial heat delivered through a heating pad, hot packs, paraffin wax, or a hot bath.

  - Cold delivered through ice packs or cold gel packs.

  - TENS unit (transcutaneous electrical nerve stimulation).

Educate in joint protection:

- See Education: Joint Protection Principles.

Improve function:

- **For hand OA**, the following **exercises performed 10 times per day in conjunction with education in joint protection principles** have been found to produce a statistically significant improvement in grip strength and global hand function (Stamm et al., 2002):

  1. Make a fist.

  2. Flex the proximal interphalangeal (PIP) and distal interphalangeal (DIP) joints only.

  3. Flex the metacarpophalangeal (MCP) joints while keeping the PIP and DIP joints stretched.

  4. Touch the tip of each finger with the tip of the thumb while keeping each finger flexed.

  5. Spread the fingers as far as possible with the hand lying flat on a table.

  6. Push each finger in the direction of the thumb with the hand lying flat on a table.

  7. Touch the MCP joint with the tip of the thumb.

  - Skilled clinical judgment should be used in prescribing specific exercises and number of repetitions.

CONDITIONS

- Create a **specialized therapeutic home exercise program** that works within the patient's pain-free ROM, does not put stress on the joints, and does not cause lasting (1–2 h) pain post workout. Program should include a low-impact aerobic component, or therapist can encourage participation in classes through assisted living facility (ALF) or in the community.

- Prescribe and grade or adapt **therapeutic activity** based on hobbies and interests.

- See Conditions: Hand Injury and Impairment for further information on OA of hand.

- **TheraPutty and resistance bands must be used with caution** to avoid compromising joint stability or increasing pain.

Occupation-based intervention/activity of daily living (ADL) retraining examples:

- The occupational therapist (OT) facilitates a meal preparation activity for a patient who complains of pain in bilateral hands due to OA. The patient is observed using a pinch grip to retrieve cookware, placing stress on thumb and smaller joints of fingers. She is educated in joint protection using both hands placed underneath a large bowl, keeping as much contact with the entire hand as possible in order to distribute weight evenly across joints of wrists and hands. The OT provides tools for the patient to trial including kitchen shears, a rocker knife, Dycem jar opener, and utensils with built-up handles. The patient complains of pain when attempting to use the kitchen shears and Dycem jar opener. Thus the OT recommends electric devices, including a food processor/chopper and an electric can and jar opener instead. Information is provided for acquiring adaptive equipment including recommendation of foam pipe insulation to be placed around existing utensils as a more affordable alternative to purchasing adaptive utensils with built up handles.

- A patient reports pain in his shoulder during activities that require him to reach overhead. The OT assesses pain-free range of shoulder flexion, which is found to be

0°–120°. The OT facilitates an organizing activity in which frequently used items in kitchen cupboards, pantry, and bedroom closet are moved to be within easy reach. Physical cues are given to ensure he avoids shoulder flexion beyond 120°. The patient learns to work within his pain-free ROM in order to maintain joint integrity while also preserving his current ROM.

OTHER CONSIDERATIONS

- **For manual muscle testing, ensure that pressure is applied in the pain-free range**. If the patient is unable to tolerate any pressure, then functional strength/ROM testing may be used as a substitute. For weak or painful hands, the bulb of a blood pressure cuff can be used to measure force in millimeters of mercury.

- Hand function and prehensile patterns can be evaluated by assessing ability to **complete common functional tasks** such as buttoning a shirt, opening a bottle, writing, or managing utensils.

- **Avoid using pulleys** to prevent injury.

- The OT can recommend the patient discuss **joint replacement or a cortisone shot** with the primary MD or orthopedist, depending on the severity of the condition.

PROVIDING CLIENT-CENTERED CARE:

- Use of adaptive equipment (AE) as a compensatory measure is central to the practice of OT. The utilization of AE is beneficial across most conditions; however, some patients may struggle to acquire the recommended equipment due to cognitive deficits or financial hardship. Providing client-centered care includes taking into consideration these limitations and assisting the patient with acquiring equipment. For example, the OT may enlist the help of a patient advocate such as an involved family member or provide community resources for gently used equipment.

CONDITIONS

26

Pain

PAIN

Acute pain is the response to an identifiable underlying pathological issue with the purpose of alerting the individual to injury. This type of pain generally responds well to medical and therapeutic intervention, subsiding as the condition improves. Conversely, chronic pain often does not serve a biological purpose and is typically more difficult to alleviate. It may be caused by remaining pain signals from a previous injury or illness, or by a chronic condition such as arthritis, low back pain, or fibromyalgia.

ASSESSMENT

VERBAL AND COGNITIVELY INTACT PATIENTS:

- Verbal Rating Scale
- 0–10 Numeric Pain Intensity Scale
- Wong Baker Faces Scale

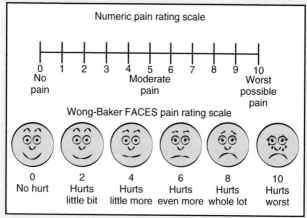

- The Brief Pain Inventory can be beneficial in determining how pain impacts various areas of the patient's life.

NONVERBAL OR COGNITIVELY IMPAIRED PATIENTS:

- Abbey Pain Assessment Scale
- Observation of pain-related behaviors such as guarded movement, facial grimacing, and protective posturing.

INTERVENTION

- When a person experiences pain, it's common for her to avoid physical activity and become more sedentary. However, this **inactivity can lead to muscle weakness and stiffness, which can exacerbate the pain** and cause her to become even more sedentary, leading to a cycle of pain and inactivity. To break this cycle, it's important to **encourage movement** through gentle exercise or therapeutic activities that are based on the person's interests or hobbies.

- Educate in **postural alignment** and **proper body mechanics** (see Education: Proper Body Mechanics).

- Instruct in applicable **joint protection techniques** (see Education: Joint Protection Principles).

- Guide patient through **progressive muscle relaxation** or **visualization/guided imagery.**

- Educate in principles of **energy conservation** (see Education: Energy Conservation Techniques).

- Identify and train in applicable **adaptive equipment** (see Additional Intervention: Adaptive Equipment).

THERAPEUTIC MODALITIES:

- **Superficial heat agent**: Increases blood flow bringing antibodies and nutrients to injured tissue, reduces stiffness, induces muscle relaxation, and has an analgesic effect. Beneficial for muscle and joint pain, arthritis (take caution with rheumatoid arthritis [RA]), chronic back pain, contractures, fibromyalgia, and myofascial pain.

  - **Contraindications**: Acute trauma, multiple sclerosis, deep vein thrombosis (DVT), neuropathy, tumors, acute inflammation, or edema.

- **Cryotherapy**: Reduces bleeding, inflammation, and swelling/edema, elevates pain threshold, and lessens tissue damage. Beneficial for acute injury, inflammation, arthritis, spasticity, and muscle pain. Treatment should be limited to 15 min of exposure.

  - **Contraindications**: Raynaud's, peripheral vascular disease, multiple myeloma/leukemia.

- **TENS unit** (transcutaneous electrical nerve stimulation).

  - **Contraindications:** Epilepsy, pacemaker. **Precaution:** Cancer, impaired sensation, pregnancy

- Other modalities include **therapeutic ultrasound** and **electrotherapy**, which require additional training and may require certification to administer.

PHARMACOLOGICAL INTERVENTION:

- Medications depend on the severity of the pain and typically range from aspirin, acetaminophen, or nonsteroidal antiinflammatory drugs (NSAIDs) to codeine or morphine for more intense pain. Occupational therapy (OT) intervention regarding pain medication may include patient or caregiver training in a **med management program** including the use of a medi-set. The OT should also identify and address any barriers to medication adherence, such as difficulty opening pill bottles or remembering to take medications.

Occupation-based intervention/activity of daily living (ADL) retraining examples:

- A patient with exacerbation of chronic low back pain states that his condition has prevented him from performing cleaning duties in his home. The OT educates in core stability training through performance of basic cleaning activities including picking up objects from the floor and vacuuming. The patient is first guided in establishing safe dynamic posture through physical cueing for proper alignment with an emphasis on neutral spine and pelvis. The patient receives verbal instruction to stabilize the position by tightening the abdominal muscles approximately 20%. From this position, he is instructed in the diagonal lift and half kneel lift to retrieve items from floor and is cued to increase abdominal tension when moving or lifting heavier objects. Core stabilization is reviewed with the vacuuming task; additional physical cues are given to prevent twisting of the spine that is common with vacuuming motions. The OT demonstrates compensatory strategy of turning with whole body and isolating shoulder movements to perform the task.

- A patient with fibromyalgia reports an increase in generalized pain that has caused her to become more inactive and somewhat resistive to therapy. This sedentary behavior inadvertently causes a further increase in pain levels. In order to encourage participation with therapy, the OT leverages the patient's favorite hobby, bowling. The activity is adapted by having the patient roll a foam ball toward water bottles set up as pins. The patient then resets the "pins" while following verbal cues from the OT for proper body mechanics.

OTHER CONSIDERATIONS

- Ensure that **documentation establishes a clear link** between pain interventions and the intended improvement of occupational performance.
- A growing body of evidence supports the use of **alternative practices** such as yoga and mindful meditation as effective tools in reducing activity in parts of the brain associated with pain signals (Khan, 2018). The OT can provide information regarding community classes or look to incorporate techniques into functional activities.

PROVIDING CLIENT-CENTERED CARE:

- Pain often deters the patient from engaging in activities they deem unnecessary, such as favorite hobbies or other leisure pursuits. Discuss how pain might impact participation with such occupations and explore options for adapting these activities in order to continue engagement in a more pain-free manner.

CONDITIONS

27

Parkinson Disease

PARKINSON DISEASE

Parkinson disease (PD) is a neurodegenerative disorder impairing movement. Occupational performance is most affected by motor symptoms including tremors, rigidity, freezing, and bradykinesia (a delay in initiating and executing movement). Mobility-related activities of daily living (MR-ADL) are impacted by gait disturbances and poor postural reactions.

ASSESSMENT

Basic:

- Range of motion (ROM)
- Manual muscle testing (MMT)
- Proprioception
- Rigidity

Functional ability & mobility:

- Modified Barthel Index (MBI)
- Functional Independence measure (FIM)
- Lawton Instrumental Activities of Daily Living (IADL) Scale
- Performance Assessment of Self Care Skills (PASS)
- Timed Up and Go Test (TUG)
- Five Times Sit to Stand

Hand strength and coordination:

- Pinch and Grip Strength (Dynamometer)
- Purdue Pegboard tests

- Nine-hole Peg Test
- Finger-tapping test

Balance/fall risk:
- Berg Balance Scale (BBS)
- Tinetti Balance and Gait Assessment
- Modified Clinical Test of Sensory Interaction in Balance (CTSIB-M)

Cognitive function:
- Scales for Outcomes in Parkinson Disease-Cognition (SCOPA-COG)
- Cambridge Cognitive Assessment Revised (CAMCOG-R)
- Mini Mental State Examination (MMSE)
- Montreal Cognitive Assessment (MoCA)

Ability to live independently:
- Kohlman Evaluation of Living Skills (KELS)
- Allen Cognitive Level Screen (ACLS)

Pain:
- Verbal Rating Scale
- 0–10 Numeric Pain Intensity Scale
- Wong Baker Faces Scale
- The Brief Pain Inventory
- Observation of pain-related behaviors such as guarded movement, facial grimacing, and protective posturing.

Depression:
- The Geriatric Depression Scale (GDS)
- Beck Depression Inventory (BDI)

Quality of life:
- The Parkinson Disease Questionnaire (PDQ-39)

Comprehensive:
- MDS-Unified Parkinson Disease Rating Scale (MDS-UPDRS)

INTERVENTION

REMEDIAL TECHNIQUES:

- Train in **postural flexibility exercises** with a focus on neck/trunk extension and chest expansion to mitigate the stooped posture associated with PD. Instruct patient to monitor their posture throughout the day by checking in a mirror. Recommend lumbar support when seated.

- Establish a daily exercise program emphasizing **full ROM**.

- **Lee Silverman Voice Treatment BIG:** Evidence-based program facilitating **large movements** through full ROM in order to slow the development of motor control abnormalities associated with PD. Requires LSVT training and certification.

- **Parkinson Wellness Recovery (PWR):** A holistic-style program offering classes directly to patients as well as workshops and certification for clinicians. Exercises are performed with **large amplitude, high effort, and attention to action** and are carried out in multiple positions.

COMPENSATORY TECHNIQUES:

- **Rhythmic Auditory Stimulation (RAS):** The provision of **rhythmic cues** (music, metronome, etc.) to signal the **initiation and cadence of movement**, improving gait and upper extremity function. Patients can also be instructed to count or sing internally for self-cueing.

- **Timing:** Educate patients in timing activities for when Levodopa/Carbidopa is most effective.

- **Orthostatic hypotension:** Educate in **pausing with positional changes**, pumping extremities prior to standing, staying hydrated, and monitoring blood pressure (BP).

- **Instruct patient in the "5s" method** when freezing occurs:

  - Stop → Stand up tall → Sigh, take a deep breath → Shift weight side to side → Start over with a big step.

- Train in **safe turning technique** using wide turns with sidestepping. Instruct in shifting weight to one foot and then leading the turn with the unweighted foot, instead of turning with upper body first.

- Train in **rocking motion** to rise from a chair.
- Educate in **fall prevention** strategies including environmental modifications (see Education: Fall Prevention).
- **ADL Modifications/adaptive equipment:**
  - **Feeding:** Weighted cuff, swivel fork/spoon, Readi Steadi Anti-Tremor Glove, Liftware.
  - **Dressing:** Velcro closure, magnetic buttons, dressing stick, button hook.
  - **Bathing:** Shower chair/transfer bench, grab bars, modify to walk-in shower if possible, long-handled sponge, caregiver training in providing assist.
  - **Toileting:** Riser, bedside commode, grab bars, handheld bidet.
  - ADL retraining with integration of **energy conservation techniques** (see Education: Energy Conservation Techniques).

LATE STAGE:

- **Dysphagia:** See Conditions: Dysphagia, Speech-Language Pathology (SLP) referral may be indicated.
- **Dementia:** See Conditions: Alzheimer Disease/Dementia.
- **Rigidity/stiffness/contractures:** Train caregivers in active or passive range of motion (A/PROM) as appropriate.

Occupation-based intervention/ADL retraining examples:

- A patient reports difficulty walking to the bathroom due to episodes of freezing and also poor balance while washing face at sink. The occupational therapist (OT) uses rhythmic auditory stimulation in the form of a metronome app and places painters tape on the floor at intervals of 2.5 feet to facilitate appropriate step length to bathroom. As a compensatory strategy to improve balance, the OT instructs the patient to brace against the sink with his body and nondominant upper extremity while washing face using a sponge in the dominant hand.
- The OT facilitates a seated dressing activity using principles of amplitude training. The patient is verbally cued to use large, effortful movements and is given

CONDITIONS

"targets" (therapist places hand to be tapped at the end of patient's full range of motion). This may include having patient thread upper extremity through sleeve flexing shoulder 170° to tap therapist's hand.

OTHER CONSIDERATIONS

- If symptoms appear to be worsening or poorly managed, the OT should **report this information to the patient's neurologist and referring MD** as carbidopa and/or levodopa may need adjusting.

- Due to a serotonergic deficit, patients with PD frequently present with depression (Ho et al., 2021); thus, **a basic depression screening may be appropriate**. Results should be reported to the referring MD.

- Driving can be particularly dangerous as the disease progresses due to the cognitive demand of processing large amounts of information efficiently, as well as the need for quick and accurate motor responses. **Driver safety concerns should be discussed with patient and family.**

- **Community resource: Rock Stead Boxing** is a nonprofit organization offering noncontact boxing exercise classes in gyms around the country. Exercises are adapted from boxing drills and promote improved gross motor movement, balance, core strength, and rhythm.

PROVIDING CLIENT-CENTERED CARE:

- Interdisciplinary communication is an important aspect of client-centered care. In the case of neurodivergent patients, it can be particularly beneficial to share specific treatment strategies to which the patient responds well. This may be in the form of certain verbal and physical cues or stimulation (e.g., music, metronome, or counting).

28

Pressure Ulcers

PRESSURE ULCERS (BED SORES, DECUBITUS ULCERS)

A pressure ulcer is a localized injury to the skin (stage 1) and underlying structures (stages 2–4). It is typically the result of prolonged pressure causing restricted blood flow and, in some cases, necrosis of the tissue. Sores usually form over bony prominences with the most common site being the sacral region.

STAGES

- **Stage 1:** Skin is closed, appears red, and does not blanch.
- **Stage 2:** Partial-thickness loss of dermis, skin is broken or looks like a blister filled with fluid and is painful.
- **Stage 3:** Full-thickness tissue loss with fat visible. Sores may not be painful due to impaired sensation at this stage.
- **Stage 4:** Full-thickness tissue loss with exposure of bone, tendon, and muscle. Patient is at risk of osteomyelitis (infection of bone) and sepsis (infection of blood).

PREVENTION

- Encourage **frequent movement** (walking or weight shifts).
- **Protect skin** from shearing, moisture, and heat.
- **Change soiled briefs** immediately.
- Perform **frequent skin checks**.
- Ensure adequate **nutrition and hydration**.
- Use **proper transfer techniques** to avoid shearing.
- **Check that the primary place of sitting is a good fit** and allows the patient the **ability to offload** if s/he is

CONDITIONS

able, **does not promote sacral sitting**, and has adequate lateral support and lower extremity support **so feet do not dangle.**

POSITIONING:

- If wheelchair-bound, **pressure reliefs** should be performed **every 30–60 min for approximately 30–60 s** to promote blood flow to sacral region and reduce risk of skin breakdown. Standing to perform pressure relief is ideal; however, if standing is not an option, patient and caregiver should be trained in:

  - **Lateral weight shifts:** Leaning to one side, push off the armrest to fully offload weight from one side of bottom. Repeat for other side.

  - **Forward weight shifts:** Leaning forward, bring weight off of bottom.

  - **Wheelchair push-ups:** If patient has adequate strength, s/he may push up on armrests to lift bottom off of cushion.

  - If unable to perform pressure reliefs (and if not in tilt-in-space), the patient should be **transferred to bed after approximately 1 h of upright sitting.**

- In bed, the patient should be **repositioned every 2 h** with special care to protect skin covering bony prominences, including:

  - Sacral region, spine, heels, ankles, scapulae, elbows, knees, wrists, ears, back of head, and temporal region.

- Pillows or wedges should be used to prop **at least 30° for right and left side-lying** to ensure adequate circulation.

- Pillows should be used **under head, arms, between knees, ankles, and to float heels.**

INTERVENTION

PATIENT AND CAREGIVER TRAINING:

- **Position patient off of wound** at all times.

- Review/educate in **positioning techniques and pressure relief/turning schedule** with caregivers.

- Review/educate in **immediate change of soiled briefs** and wet sheets to prevent skin breakdown.
- Ensure that **turning sheets** are being used to reposition patient in order to minimize shearing force.

PRESSURE RELIEVING DEVICES:

- Air cell/ROHO cushion
  - Pressure should be checked daily and adjusted as needed
- Gel cushion
- Waffle cushion
- Alternating pressure pad
- Foam or gel mattress overlay
- Low air loss mattress
- Tilt-in-space wheel chair
- Heel protector boot
- Wedges/pillows
- Bed rails or trapeze to assist with turning
  - Depending on the setting, bed rails may be considered a restraint and therefore prohibited

FACTORS TO CONSIDER WHEN CHOOSING A DEVICE:

- Stage of pressure ulcer
- Level of mobility/ability to weight shift
- Cognition
- Prior history of sores
- Continence status
- Braden Scale score

Occupation-based intervention/activity of daily living (ADL) retraining example:

- A patient and a caregiver are trained in the changing of an incontinent brief in a skilled nursing facility (SNF) setting. The patient has a history of prolonged immobilization and current stage 2 pressure ulcer. The staff had been using slide board transfer, but the occupational therapist (OT) now recommends use of

CONDITIONS

mechanical lift to avoid shearing force that may occur with the slide board. The OT ensures proper use of mechanical lift to transfer the patient from tilt-in-space to bed. Once in bed, a turning sheet is used to prop the patient on her side. She is encouraged to participate by holding onto the half rail, helping to keep herself turned on her side while the OT and caregiver complete peri-care. The caregiver is reminded to check for soiled briefs frequently and the patient is instructed to alert staff if she is aware of an incontinent episode. The OT educates the patient and caregiver in repositioning to 30° side-lying and use of pillows to protect bony prominences. The OT reviews the turning schedule with the caregiver and instructs the patient to remind staff if repositioning does not occur in a timely manner.

OTHER CONSIDERATIONS

- Although a nutrition screening will likely be performed by skilled nursing (SN), OT can (as part of the interdisciplinary team) **endorse adequate protein intake and hydration.**

- The OT can inquire regarding **insurance coverage** for pressure-relieving devices and submit a letter of justification if required.

DELIVERING CLIENT-CENTERED CARE:

- Patients diagnosed with pressure ulcers are often immobile and require assistance with care. When a patient is cognitively intact to do so, s/he should be empowered to direct her/his own care. This not only helps to ensure proper management of the condition but also allows the patient to be an active participant in her/his care rather than a passive recipient. Education is a fundamental component of client-centered care and helps to provide the patient with a sense of agency, which can be invaluable when depending on others for care.

29

Respiratory Conditions

RESPIRATORY CONDITIONS

For chronic obstructive pulmonary disease (COPD) patients, be sure to find/request O_2 parameters prior to starting care, as the target O_2 saturation for this population is often 88–92%.

Respiratory conditions affect the respiratory system, which includes the organs and tissues involved in breathing, such as the lungs, bronchi, trachea, larynx, and nasal passages. They can be acute or chronic and can range from mild to severe. Common respiratory conditions include COPD, asthma, pneumonia, emphysema, chronic bronchitis, pleural effusion, and lung cancer. Activity of daily living (ADL) performance is generally compromised by dyspnea and decreased activity tolerance. Additionally, reliance on upper thoracic/intercostal and accessory muscles for breathing, rather than the diaphragm, causes difficulty performing activities involving the upper extremities.

ASSESSMENT

Endurance:

- 6 Minute Walk Test (6MWT)

Functional ability & mobility:

- Modified Barthel Index (MBI)
- Canadian Occupational Performance Measure (COPM)
- Timed Up and Go Test (TUG)
- Five Times Sit to Stand

Perceived exertion:

- Borg Rate of Perceived Exertion (RPE) Scale (see Conditions: Cardiovascular Disease for scale)

INTERVENTION

- **Early mobilization** in acute care/intensive care unit (ICU).

- Educate in **ventilation strategies**:
  - Pursed lip breathing
  - Diaphragmatic breathing (Hobbs (2016))
  - Huff coughing: Basic airway clearance technique
  - Active cycle breathing to clear mucus from the lungs
- Educate in the importance of **posture** in order for diaphragm to flatten, producing expansion of thoracic cavity and lungs.
- Train in **synchronizing breath and movement** in accordance with intra-abdominal pressure:
  - Inhale during the lighter portion of the task and exhale during the strenuous portion of the task.
- Establish a **low-endurance cardiopulmonary exercise program** including stretching and strengthening of the upper body.
- Educate in **awareness of dyspnea** while performing activities:
  - Borg RPE Scale
- **Positioning**: Advise laying on side with head elevated (lateral recumbent position) or on back with head of bed elevated 15°–45° and place a cushion under knees.
- Recommend **ADL modifications and adaptive equipment** (see Additional Intervention: Adaptive Equipment).
- Train in **energy conservation techniques** (see Education: Energy Conservation Techniques).
- Train in **proper body mechanics** (see Education: Proper Body Mechanics).
- Assess for **environmental or occupational irritants** and recommend ways to avoid pollutants, such as use of a High Efficiency Particulate Air (HEPA) air filter.
- Educate in **supplemental O_2 use**:
  - Train in safe mobility-related activities of daily living (MR-ADL) while managing O_2 tubing throughout the home.
  - Ensure O_2 use during shower.

- **Decrease feelings of anxiety** associated with shortness of breath:
  - Relaxation techniques, deep breathing, sleep hygiene.

Occupation-based intervention/ADL retraining examples:

- A patient with COPD is retrained in safe seated shower using techniques to decrease cardiac workload. The occupational therapist (OT) first educates in setup utilizing principles of energy conservation, including use of tub transfer bench, decreasing water temperature to warm rather than hot, and proper ventilation (turning on bathroom fan and leaving door and window open). During shower, the patient is cued to take frequent rest breaks and minimize overhead activity; tripod posture is used to wash hair, and a terrycloth bathrobe with hood is used to dry hair and body.

- A patient with asthma becomes short of breath (SOB) with moderate exertion. The OT guides patient through a session of tidying up his room including making his bed. The OT first shows the patient the Borg's Rating of Perceived Exertion (RPE) Scale with scores from 6 (no exertion) to 20 (maximal exertion) and requests that the patient attempt to keep rating from light to moderate (10–11) in order to avoid becoming SOB. The patient is instructed in abdominal breathing and proper dynamic posture (neutral spine and pelvis), which he performs in front of mirror for visual feedback. The OT demonstrates coiling O_2 tubing and holding it against the walker to prevent tripping/falling. He is trained in use of long-handled reacher to retrieve items from floor and is directed to take frequent, short rest breaks. To make the bed, he is instructed in synchronizing breath with intra-abdominal pressure: exhaling while reaching down to manage bedding and inhaling when standing back up for proper thoracic expansion.

OTHER CONSIDERATIONS

- **A doctor's order may be required to check oxygen levels.** This should be checked in the chart prior to treating patient.

CONDITIONS

- It is recommended that patients with COPD receive a **flu and pneumococcal vaccine** yearly. Studies have found that vaccination decreases pneumonia diagnoses, hospitalizations, and cardiac events in this population (Udell et al., 2013).

- Patients who are still smoking should be provided with information on **cessation programs.**

- Encourage compliance with Bilevel Positive Airway Pressure **(BiPAP)**/Continuous Positive Airway Pressure **(CPAP)** if prescribed by MD.

- **Chest physical therapy (CPT)** will likely be performed by the physical therapist (PT); however, in some settings the OT may educate in postural drainage or perform percussion to loosen mucus in the lungs.

PROVIDING CLIENT-CENTERED CARE:

- Becoming SOB, a common symptom of respiratory conditions, can cause patients to feel anxious or distressed. Showing concern for, and attempting to alleviate any physical or emotional discomfort during treatment is an important element of client-centered care (Tzelepis et al., 2015). In addition to the interventions listed above, the OT can apply principles of therapeutic use of self to help the patient feel more at ease during activity.

30

Spinal Cord Injury

A spinal cord injury (SCI) is damage to the spinal cord that results in a loss of function, sensation, or movement. The severity of an SCI depends on the location and extent of the damage. It is important to recognize that the functional levels associated with spinal cord injury should be interpreted with caution, as they may not capture the full extent of an individual's abilities and may not fully account for the wide range of factors that can affect functional capacity. As such, while these levels can provide a useful framework for understanding the general impact of spinal cord injury on physical function, they should not be viewed as an absolute measure of a person's ability to perform activities of daily living or engage in meaningful occupations.

SPINAL CORD INJURY (SCI)			
SPINAL CORD LEVELS	MUSCLES	ACTION	TYPICAL FUNCTIONAL LEVEL
C1–C3	Sternocleidomastoid, rectus capitis, longus colli and capitis	Neck flexion, extension, lateral flexion, and rotation	• Often fatal • Dependent for all care • Ventilator dependent • Potential to drive adaptive power chair • 24-h care
C4	Upper trapezius, diaphragm, spinalis cervicis	Scapular elevation, inspiration	• Dependent for all care • Potential for independent respiration • 24-h care

SPINAL CORD LEVELS	MUSCLES	ACTION	TYPICAL FUNCTIONAL LEVEL
C5	Deltoid, rhomboids, supraspinatus infraspinatus, teres minor, subscapularis (partial rotator cuff innervation), biceps, brachialis, brachioradialis, serratus anterior (partial innervation)	Scapular abduction, adduction, shoulder flexion, extension, abduction, weak elbow flexion, and forearm supination	• Self-feeds with adaptive device such as U-cuff • Min/mod assistance with upper body activities of daily living (ADLs) • Max assistance with lower body ADLs • 10 h/day caregiver
C6	Full innervation of rotator cuff, clavicular pectoralis, biceps, extensor carpi radialis longus and brevis, serratus anterior (full innervation), latissimus dorsi (partial innervation)	Scapular upward rotation, shoulder internal/external rotation, shoulder adduction, horizontal adduction, strong elbow flexion, wrist extension/tenodesis	• Modified independent with upper body ADLs • Minimum assistance with lower body ADLs • Wrist extension: able to grasp using tenodesis function • Limited bed mobility • Drives with hand controls • Able to participate with transfers • Pushes manual chair • 0–6 h/day caregiver
C7	Latissimus dorsi, sternal pectoralis, triceps, flexor carpi radialis, flexor digitorum superficialis, extensor digitorum, extensor pollicis	Strong elbow extension, forearm pronation, wrist flexion, weak finger flexion, finger/thumb extension	• Independent wheelchair level transfer • Modified independent for most ADLs • 0–2 h/day caregiver

SPINAL CORD LEVELS	MUSCLES	ACTION	TYPICAL FUNCTIONAL LEVEL
C8	Flexor carpi ulnaris, extensor carpi ulnaris, flexor pollicis longus and brevis, abductor pollicis longus, opponens pollicis, adductor pollicis, flexor digitorum profundus, and superficialis	Strong wrist extension with ulnar and radial deviation, thumb flexion, abduction/adduction/opposition, strong finger flexion, flexion of metacarpophalangeals (MCPs) with interphalangeal (IP) extension	• Modified independent for all ADLs and most IADLs • Potential to live independently in the community
T1–T6	Abductor pollicis brevis, dorsal and palmar Interossei, erector spinae of upper back, upper intercostals	Thumb abduction, finger abduction, IP abduction, MCP joint flexion with IP joint extension, thoracic spine extension	• Independent for all ADLs and instrumental activities of daily living (IADLs) • Able to utilize standing frame
T7–T12	Abdominals, quadratus lumborum (partial)	Stable thoracic muscles, functional intercostals, trunk flexion and rotation, partial pelvic floor	• Stands with full leg brace • Potential for ambulation with bilateral upper extremity support

SPINAL CORD LEVELS	MUSCLES	ACTION	TYPICAL FUNCTIONAL LEVEL
L1–L2	Quadratus lumborum (full), iliopsoas	Hip flexion	• Good sitting balance • Ambulation with device
L3–L4	Lower erector spinae, quadriceps, hip flexors, hamstring (partial), anterior tibialis	Lumbar extension, knee flexion/extension, weak ankle dorsiflexion	• Ambulation with braces only

Data from Pendleton, H., & Schultz-Krohn, W. (2017). *Pedretti's occupational therapy: Practice skills for physical dysfunction (occupational therapy skills for physical dysfunction (Pedretti))* (8th ed.). Mosby (Morgan (n.d.)).

ASSESSMENT

Basic:

- Range of motion (ROM)
- Manual muscle testing (MMT)
- Sensation
  - Semmes-Weinstein Monofilament Test
- Proprioception
- Tone
- Bowel and bladder
- Autonomic regulation/orthostatic hypotension

Functional activity & mobility:

- Spinal Cord Independence Measure III (SCIM)
- Modified Barthel Index (MBI)
- Functional Independence Measure (FIM)
- Canadian Occupational Performance Measure (COPM)

- Walking Index for Spinal Cord Injury II (WISCI II)
- Six Minute Walk Test (6MWT)
- Wheelchair Skills Test

Upper extremity function:

- Capabilities of Upper Extremity Questionnaire (CUE-Q)
- Sollerman Hand Function Test
- Jebsen Taylor Hand Functioning Test

Balance/fall risk:

- Berg Balance Scale (BBS)

Pain:

- Verbal Rating Scale
- 0–10 Numeric Pain Intensity Scale
- Wong Baker Faces Scale
- The Brief Pain Inventory
- Observation of pain-related behaviors such as guarded movement, facial grimacing, and protective posturing.

ASIA exam

- The International Standards for Neurological Classification of Spinal Cord Injury (ISNCSCI), more commonly known as the ASIA Exam is a standardized, sensory and motor assessment that also determines the completeness of the injury.

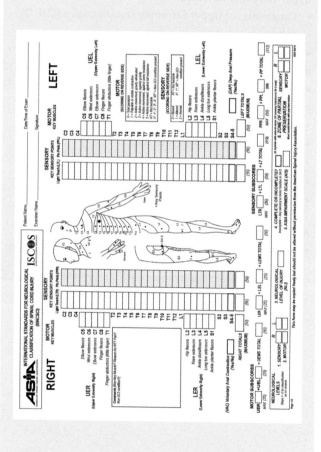

Muscle Function Grading

0 = Total paralysis
1 = Palpable or visible contraction
2 = Active movement, full range of motion (ROM) with gravity eliminated
3 = Active movement, full ROM against gravity
4 = Active movement, full ROM against gravity and moderate resistance in a muscle specific position
5 = (normal) active movement, full ROM against gravity and full resistance in a functional muscle position expected from an otherwise unimpaired person
NT = Not testable (i.e. due to immobilization, severe pain such that the patient cannot be graded, amputation of limb, or contracture of > 50% of the normal ROM)
0*, 1*, 2*, 3*, 4*, NT* = Non-SCI condition present *

Sensory Grading

0 = Absent 1 = Altered, either decreased/impaired sensation or hypersensitivity
2 = Normal NT = Not testable

0*, 1*, NT* = Non-SCI condition present *

Note: Abnormal motor and sensory scores should be tagged with a '' to indicate an impairment due to a non-SCI condition. The non-SCI condition should be explained in the comments box together with information about how the score is rated for classification purposes (at least normal / not normal for classification).

When to Test Non-Key Muscles:

In a patient with an apparent AIS B classification, non-key muscle functions more than 3 levels below the motor level on each side should be tested to most accurately classify the injury (differentiate between AIS B and C).

Movement	Root level
Shoulder: Flexion, extension, abduction, adduction, internal and external rotation Elbow: Supination	C5
Elbow: Pronation Wrist: Flexion	C6
Finger: Flexion at proximal joint, extension Thumb: Flexion, extension and abduction in plane of thumb	C7
Finger: Flexion at MCP joint Thumb: Opposition, adduction and abduction perpendicular to palm	C8
Finger: Abduction of the index finger	T1
Hip: Adduction	L2
Hip: External rotation	L3
Hip: Extension, abduction, internal rotation Knee: Flexion Ankle: Inversion and eversion Toe: MP and IP extension	L4
Hallux and Toe: DIP and PIP flexion and abduction	L5
Hallux: Adduction	S1

ASIA Impairment Scale (AIS)

A = Complete. No sensory or motor function is preserved in the sacral segments S4-5.

B = Sensory Incomplete. Sensory but not motor function is preserved below the neurological level and includes the sacral segments S4-5 (light touch or pin prick at S4-5 or deep anal pressure) AND no motor function is preserved more than three levels below the motor level on either side of the body.

C = Motor Incomplete. Motor function is preserved at the most caudal sacral segments for voluntary anal contraction (VAC) OR the patient meets the criteria for sensory incomplete status (sensory function preserved at the most caudal sacral segments S4-5 by LT, PP or DAP), and has some sparing of motor function more than three levels below the ipsilateral motor level on either side of the body.
(This includes key or non-key muscle functions to determine motor incomplete status.) For AIS C – less than half of key muscle functions below the single NLI have a muscle grade ≥ 3.

D = Motor Incomplete. Motor incomplete status as defined above, with at least half (half or more) of key muscle functions below the single NLI having a muscle grade ≥ 3.

E = Normal. If sensation and motor function as tested with the ISNCSCI are graded as normal in all segments, and the patient had prior deficits, then the AIS grade is E. Someone without an initial SCI does not receive an AIS grade.

Using ND: To document the sensory, motor and NLI levels, the ASIA Impairment Scale grade, and/or the zone of partial preservation (ZPP) when they are unable to be determined based on the examination results.

[ASIA / ISCOS logo]

AMERICAN SPINAL INJURY ASSOCIATION

INTERNATIONAL STANDARDS FOR NEUROLOGICAL CLASSIFICATION OF SPINAL CORD INJURY

ISCOS
INTERNATIONAL SPINAL CORD SOCIETY

Page 2/2

Steps in Classification

The following order is recommended for determining the classification of individuals with SCI.

1. Determine sensory levels for right and left sides.
The sensory level is the most caudal, intact dermatome for both pin prick and light touch sensation.

2. Determine motor levels for right and left sides.
Defined by the lowest key muscle function that has a grade of at least 3 (on supine testing), providing the key muscle functions represented by segments above that level are judged to be intact (graded as a 5).
Note: in regions where there is no myotome to test, the motor level is presumed to be the same as the sensory level, if testable motor function above that level is also normal.

3. Determine the neurological level of injury (NLI).
This refers to the most caudal segment of the cord with intact sensation and antigravity (3 or more) muscle function strength, provided that there is normal (intact) sensory and motor function rostrally respectively.
The NLI is the most cephalad of the sensory and motor levels determined in steps 1 and 2.

4. Determine whether the injury is Complete or Incomplete.
(i.e. absence or presence of sacral sparing)
If voluntary anal contraction = No AND all S4-5 sensory scores = 0
AND deep anal pressure = No, then injury is Complete.
Otherwise, injury is Incomplete.

5. Determine ASIA Impairment Scale (AIS) Grade.

Is injury Complete? If YES, AIS=A

NO ↓

Is injury Motor Complete? If YES, AIS=B

NO ↓ (No=voluntary anal contraction OR motor function more than three levels below the motor level on a given side, if the patient has sensory incomplete classification)

Are at least half (half or more) of the key muscles below the neurological level of injury graded 3 or better?

NO ↓   YES ↓
AIS=C   AIS=D

If sensation and motor function is normal in all segments, AIS=E
Note: AIS E is used in follow up testing when an individual with a documented SCI has recovered normal function. If at initial testing no deficits are found, the individual is neurologically intact and the ASIA Impairment Scale does not apply.

6. Determine the zone of partial preservation (ZPP).
The ZPP is used only in injuries with absent motor (no VAC) OR sensory function (no DAP, no LT and no PP sensation) in the lowest sacral segments S4-5, and refers to those dermatomes and myotomes caudal to the sensory and motor levels that remain partially innervated. With sacral sparing of sensory function, the sensory ZPP is not applicable and therefore "NA" is recorded in the block of the worksheet. Accordingly, if VAC is present, the motor ZPP is not applicable and is noted as "NA".

Trauma RSS. (American Spinal Injury Association: International Standards for Neurological Classification of Spinal Cord Injury, revised 2019; Richmond, VA.)

CONDITIONS

INTERVENTION

- Train in **upright tolerance** and **prevention of orthostatic hypotension**.
- **Spasticity/contracture management** and prevention:
  - Positioning, stretching, splinting
- Patient education in managing **decreased vital capacity**:
  - Glossopharyngeal breathing
  - Intermittent positive pressure breathing
  - Continuous Positive Airway Pressure (CPAP)/Bilevel Positive Airway Pressure (BiPAP)
  - Effective cough
- **Prevention of pressure ulcers** (see Conditions: Pressure Ulcers)
- Educate in techniques to facilitate **tenodesis function**:
  - When performing range of motion program: Wrist extension should only occur with finger flexion. Finger extension should only occur with wrist flexion.
  - Instruct patient to prop upper body weight through arms with hands in fisted position rather than using an open hand (such as when leaning on bed/mat or when transferring). Using an open hand stretches the finger flexors and prevents development of tenodesis function.
  - Tenodesis splint.
- Management of **neurogenic bowel/bladder**:
  - Bowel program: Manual removal, digital stimulation, suppository, enema, medication.
  - Catheterization/regular voiding.
  - Urinary tract infection (UTI) prevention.
- Prescribe **adaptive equipment (AE)/durable medical equipment (DME)**, assist with attaining, and train in safe use. This equipment may include:
  - Wheelchair/seating system, transfer equipment such as lifts or boards, respiratory equipment, tools for self-care and feeding, and positioning devices. Occupational therapist (OT) should also recommend home and car modifications.

- Prescribe any **assistive technology,** assist with attaining, and train in safe use. This equipment may include:
  - Environmental control units, communication devices, emergency call systems.
- **Temperature control**:
  - Avoid extreme temperatures
  - Prepare with layers
  - Avoid long exposure to heat/sun
  - Stay hydrated
- **Autonomic dysreflexia**:
  - Signs/symptoms: Sudden onset of headache, elevated BP, slow pulse, flushed face.
  - If suspected: Sit patient upright, check for noxious stimuli (full bladder, fecal impaction, kinked catheter, tight clothing).
  - Prevention: Educate patient and caregiver in preventing noxious stimuli and in being aware of signs and symptoms.
  - Ensure regular bowel and bladder routine as distended bladder or rectum are common causes of autonomic dysreflexia.
- Sexual dysfunction:
  - Oral medication
  - Vacuum therapy
  - Penile injections/implant

Occupation-based intervention/ADL retraining example:

- A patient with a newly acquired C6 spinal cord injury (SCI) has been experiencing episodes of orthostatic hypotension (OH) in the mornings. The OT plans to address OH as well as his goal to use his cell phone independently. In supine, the OT places an abdominal binder and compression stockings on the patient, then raises the head of the bed to 30°. The OT explains the benefits of compression garments and slow positional changes in preventing OH. While allowing time for blood pressure to acclimate to positional change, OT creates a lap holder for cell phone by placing a Velcro strap around the patient's leg. Double-sided tape is used to adhere a second piece of Velcro to the back of the cell phone, which is then placed securely onto the patient's leg strap. A U-cuff with stylus in placed on the patient's hand. He is then instructed to raise the head of bed to 45° at which point he is able to access his phone. With instruction for use of stylus, the patient is able to operate phone. The patient continues to slowly raise head, being aware of any signs or symptoms of OH until he is in an upright position.

OTHER CONSIDERATIONS

- In the acute care setting, prior to evaluation, the OT must have **clear orders regarding allowed movement** which depends on the patient's spinal stability.

- Medicare, Medicaid, or private health insurance may **cover some durable medical equipment (DME).** The OT can assist with acquiring equipment and submit necessary paperwork justifying need.

- Other **psychosocial factors** that should be considered when treating a patient with SCI include
  - Loss of independence
  - Changing roles
  - Adjusting to life with a disability
  - Depression

PROVIDING CLIENT-CENTERED CARE:

- In many cases the physical impairments caused by a SCI are life-altering. As a result, patients generally must undergo a reconstruction of self and identity (Bhattarai et al., 2020). The OT is situated to assist the patient in facilitating continuity of the self prior to the disability with integration of the new identity through means of remedial and compensatory measures, activity modifications, assistive technology, adaptive equipment, and wheelchair seating design.

31

Traumatic Brain Injury

TRAUMATIC BRAIN INJURY

A traumatic brain injury (TBI) occurs when an external force causes damage to the brain tissue. The alteration in normal brain functioning could be mild to severe involving decreased consciousness, neurological changes, memory loss, and cognitive impairment.

ASSESSMENTS

Basic:

- Range of motion (ROM)
- Manual muscle testing (MMT)
- Sensation
  - Semmes-Weinstein Monofilament Test (SWMT)
- Motor signs
  - Decerebrate or decorticate rigidity, spasticity, myoclonus, bradykinesia, tremor, dystonia, chorea
- Bowel and bladder

Level of consciousness:

- Glasgow Coma Scale (GCS)
- Rancho Los Amigos Scale (RLAS)
- John F. Kennedy (JFK) Coma Recovery Scale Revised (CRS-R)
- Western Neuro Sensory Stimulation Profile

Cognitive function:

- Montreal Cognitive Assessment (MoCA)

CONDITIONS

- Stroop Color and Word Test (SCWT)
- The Symbol Digit Modalities Test (SDMT)

Behavioral regulation:
- Rancho Los Amigos Scale (RLAS)
- Behavioral Assessment Screening Tool (BAST)
- Neurobehavioral Rating Scale (NRS)

Functional ability & mobility:
- Disability Rating Scale (DRS)
- Functional Independence Measure with the addition of the Functional Assessment Measure for the brain injured population (FIM + FAM)
- Modified Barthel Index (MBI)
- Performance Assessment of Self Care Skills (PASS)
- Lawton Instrumental Activities of Daily Living (IADL) Scale
- Timed Up and Go Test (TUG)
- Five Times Sit to Stand

Balance/fall risk:
- Berg Balance Scale (BBS)
- Tinetti Balance and Gait Assessment
- Modified Clinical Test of Sensory Interaction in Balance (CTSIB-M)

Spasticity:
- Modified Ashworth Scale

Pain:
- Verbal Rating Scale
- 0–10 Numeric Pain Intensity Scale
- Wong Baker Faces Scale
- The Brief Pain Inventory
- Observation of pain-related behaviors such as guarded movement, facial grimacing, and protective posturing.

Dysphagia:
- See Conditions: Dysphagia

Visual function:
- Homonymous hemianopsia
  - Visual Field Test
- Unilateral neglect
  - Line Bisection Test
  - Cancellation Test
  - Behavioral Inattention Test (BIT)
- Visual screening
  - See Conditions: Low Vision: Visual Screening

Ability to live independently:
- Independent Living Scale (ILS)
- Kohlman Evaluation of Living Skills (KELS)
- Allen Cognitive Level Screen (ACLS)

Supervision needed for safety:
- Supervision Rating Scale (SRS)

Depression:
- Beck Depression Inventory (BDI)

Quality of life:
- Quality of Life after Brain Injury (QOLIBRI)

Comprehensive:
- National Institutes of Health Toolbox Cognition Battery (NIHTB-CB)
- Neurobehavioral Functioning Inventory (NFI)

INTERVENTION

MODERATE TO SEVERE IMPAIRMENT:

Positioning:
- **Semi-prone or side lying** provides sensory input while normalizing tone.
  - Assistive positioning supports include **pillows and wedges**.
- Supine may elicit extensor tone and, in the case of abnormal posture, is typically avoided.

CONDITIONS

Splinting:

- As patients typically present with flexion of the upper extremities, splints that place wrist and hands in **reflex-inhibiting positions, such as an antispasticity splint or a resting hand splint,** are generally recommended.

- A **cone** can be utilized to maintain thumb web space and prevent skin breakdown.

- **Serial casting** may be indicated for contractures that do not respond to splinting.

ROM program:

- Passive range of motion (PROM) with slow, sustained end range hold should be **performed daily** to treat/prevent contractures.

Seating:

- **Pelvis must be in a neutral position** or with a slight anterior tilt and evenly positioned for equal weight distribution through both buttocks (one side should not be elevated or retracted).

- A **solid seat and lumbar support** are required for proper positioning of pelvis.

- A **solid back insert or a firm contoured back** is necessary to maintain alignment of the spine.

- A **wedged seat insert** for slight hip flexion is beneficial to prevent extensor tone.

- **Lateral trunk supports** can be used to maintain midline.

- **Adductor/abductor wedges** can be used for positioning of the lower extremity (LE). Knees and ankles should be positioned to 90° and feet should rest comfortably on **foot plates**.

- A **lapboard** can be used to promote functional positioning of the upper extremity (UE).

- A **dynamic head positioning device** can be utilized in the case of poor head control; otherwise, a **contoured head rest** is typically sufficient.

- The back of the chair should be **reclined 10°–15°** for optimal positioning of head and trunk.

- Other useful equipment may include **chest-, shoulder-, or forehead-strap, lateral head supports, and leg trough.**

Behavioral management: Approach will vary greatly depending upon the patient's cognitive level.

- The therapist must first:
  - **Build trust**. Therapeutic use of self can be an effective approach in building a trusting relationship with the patient.
  - **Identify triggers** or stimuli that may be provoking.
  - Help the patient feel a **sense of control** over the environment.
  - Provide **options** from which the patient can choose.
- **Establish a schedule** and ensure adherence to a daily routine.
- Present relatively easy tasks for patient to experience a **feeling of success** and intermittently add in more challenging tasks.
- Apply **errorless** learning technique (see Additional Intervention: ADL/IADL Retraining Techniques).
- **Terminate activities** if the patient becomes frustrated.
- Ensure that the patient is able to **express his or her needs**. Explore alternative communication options if the patient is non-verbal or has difficulty expressing needs.

Sensory stimulation:

- **All senses should be stimulated** to heighten arousal and improve responsiveness to the external environment.
- Therapists should collaborate with family regarding **meaningful objects** (visual/tactile), **music preference** (auditory), and **familiar scents** (olfactory), such as regularly used shampoo.
- The **gustatory system** can be stimulated through the use of a cotton swab against the mouth containing different flavors.

CONDITIONS

Occupation-based intervention/ADL retraining example:

- The occupational therapist (OT) incorporates a painting session with the patient's PROM program to simultaneously facilitate fine motor (FM) control. The patient presents with flexion pattern of the right upper extremity (RUE). The OT performs gentle ROM of RUE and places a paintbrush in the patient's hand, using hand over hand to facilitate the proper prehensile pattern. The wrist is held at end range in slight extension for positioning against the easel.

MILD TO MODERATE IMPAIRMENT:

Gross and fine motor:

- Engage patient in activities that promote motor patterns, balance, endurance, coordination, and strength.

Cognition:

- **Attention processing training** (APT) is a structured program that consists of a progression of tasks from simple to complex which increase in attention demand.

- **Restorative memory approaches** may include word list recall, paragraph listening, and mnemonic strategies.

- **External cues** such as calendars, clocks, the day's agenda, and pictures of family and friends can help to orient the patient.

- **Remediation activities** can include games, puzzles, and worksheets, or could be computer based.

Routines:

- **Establish a consistent schedule** collaboratively with patient to create predictability and reduce anxiety.

ADLs:

- **Task simplification and sequencing:** Guide patient through only one step of an activity at a time, gradually increasing the complexity.

- **Grade activities** for an appropriate challenge.

- Utilize **forward and backward chaining**.

- Determine what type of **cueing** the patient responds well to such as verbal, visual, or physical cues or demonstration by therapist.

Neglect:

- Visual scanning

  - **Lighthouse technique**: An organized search pattern in which patient turns head fully scanning from left to right with conscious attention to detail.

  - **Anchoring (in environment)**: Bright-colored tape or other attention-grabbing objects placed on the affected side.

  - **Anchoring (on paper):** A mark such as a line or a number placed at the beginning or end of a sentence to indicate the starting and/or ending place.

  - **Letter cancellation:** Worksheets that facilitate scanning through the search of a particular letter or symbol amongst an array of characters.

- ADLs and other activities can be **performed in front of a mirror** to bring attention to the affected side.

- Caregiver training to approach and **talk to the patient on the affected side.**

- **Eye patching** and **prism glasses.**

Return to residence:

- **Home safety evaluation** with recommendations (see Assessment: Home Safety Eval/Checklist).

- Address **community mobility** and provide resources.

- **Determine amount of assistance needed** for ADL/IADL and provide caregiver training or community resources for obtaining caregiver.

Occupation-based intervention/ADL retraining example:

- The OT facilitates a cooking activity requiring the patient to plan, organize, and multitask. In order to transport items from fridge to counter, the OT provides a walker tray for the patient to trial. Upon observing signs of agitation, the OT grades the activity by breaking the task into smaller steps and providing hand over hand guidance in executing certain fine motor tasks.

OTHER CONSIDERATIONS

- The patient should be monitored for signs of **intracranial pressure (ICP)** including flaccidity, abnormal reflexes, vomiting, or changes in vital signs.

- As seizure disorders can arise after a TBI, therapy including **sensory stimulation and ROM should begin slowly** with close monitoring of responses.

PROVIDING CLIENT-CENTERED CARE:

- Agitation-type behaviors, such as restlessness, impulsivity, and aggression, are observed in approximately half of patients recovering from TBI (Carrier et al., 2021). Creating a safe space for the patient can help to avoid or reduce feelings of distress and anxiety. The OT can help to create this space by requesting that family bring items the patient finds comforting such as headphones, a poster, puzzles, a fidget toy, etc. The space can be set up in a corner of the room or any place that can be dedicated to the patient.

Additional Intervention

32

Types of Intervention

OCCUPATION/ACTIVITY-BASED TREATMENT IDEAS

The following are examples of activities that can be used as a medium to restore the skills necessary to perform activities of daily living/instrumental activities of daily living (ADLs/IADLs). In choosing an appropriate activity, ensure consideration of the specific deficits affecting occupational performance as well as individual interests. The following fine/gross motor activities can be carried out while sitting or standing and should be graded to provide a fitting challenge.

ACTIVITIES THAT PROMOTE FINE MOTOR SKILLS

Equipment required:

- Sort/twist nuts, bolts, and washers
- Sort/stack coins
- Polymer clay modeling
- Basic meal prep
- Sort deck of cards
- Lacing boards
- Pick up/sort small objects with clothespins or tweezers
- Lace large beads
- Games/puzzles
- Make fishing lures/tie onto line
- Remove and replace batteries and lightbulbs from flashlight
- Sanding and repainting
- Simple woodworking kit
- Painting or writing on a vertical surface

ADDITIONAL INTERVENTION

- TheraPutty
- Digiflex

Crafts:
- Origami
- Stencils
- Ribbon weaving
- Simple macrame
- Greeting cards
- No-sew tie blanket
- Make bird seed ornaments that can be hung outside the patient's window
- Pressed flowers or flower pens
- Crochet/needlework
- Jewelry making

Using items from patient's room/house:
- Unscrew and replace bottle caps of various sizes (medication bottles, hygiene products, etc.)
- Empty silverware tray, clean the tray, organize/replace silverware
- Button/unbutton clothing, threading, and hooking a belt
- Wring out washcloth/sponge
- Fold laundry
- Organize cupboard
- Write letters to family and friends

ACTIVITIES THAT PROMOTE GROSS MOTOR SKILLS, BALANCE, AND FUNCTIONAL ACTIVITY TOLERANCE

Equipment required:
- Bowling: Use empty or filled water bottles as pins
- Putt putt golf: Use cane as golf club to putt ball into mug laying on its side
- Ring toss: Cut out center of paper plates and use the outer ring to toss on water bottles placed at varying distances
- Jumbo Connect Four: Hang a sheet or tablecloth on a wall. Trace paper plates (6 rows and 7 columns) to

create 42 circles and place Velcro in the center of each circle. Adhere Velcro to the back of 42 plates (using two different colors of plates)

- Vertical match: Tape a deck of playing cards to a poster, adding a piece of Velcro to the front of each. Use a second deck with Velcro added to match the cards
- Bean bag toss: Use baggies filled with beans to toss into shoe boxes with holes cut into the lids
- Magnetic dart board
- Play catch with large ball or bat balloon with hand, paddle, or water noodle
- Planting or potting
- Obstacle course

Using items from patient's room/house:
- Basic activities of daily living (BADLs)
- Clean and organize fridge, pantry, or drawers, throwing away expired containers
- Organize closet space
- Learn basic dance steps
- Functional transfers throughout home or facility (bed, shower, toilet, wheelchair, dining room chair, etc.)
- Load, rotate, and fold laundry
- Organize closet and drawers
- Tie a resistance band in a circle, have patient step into loop (or bring over feet in sitting), work band up body and overhead. Reverse starting by bringing loop overhead and pushing it down, taking it off around feet
- Retrieve items placed at various heights around room
- Utilizing proprioceptive neuromuscular facilitation (PNF) patterns, pick items up from floor (or low surface) and place overhead (or hand items to therapist)
- Have patient adjust height of walker or wheelchair, then return it to appropriate height
- Unload and load dishwasher
- Change the sheets, make the bed

33

ADL/IADL Retraining Techniques

ACTIVITY OF DAILY LIVING/INSTRUMENTAL ACTIVITY OF DAILY LIVING (ADL/IADL) RETRAINING TECHNIQUES

GRADING: To increase or decrease the difficulty of an activity in order to provide the patient with an appropriate challenge.

BACKWARD CHAINING: Mastering an activity by learning the last step first and progressing in a backward manner. The occupational therapist (OT) completes all steps (or assists in completing steps) other than the last, which is completed by the patient. Once the patient is proficient with the last step, the OT then completes all steps other than the last two and so on until the patient is able to complete the activity independently.

FORWARD CHAINING: Mastering an activity by learning each step in sequential order. The patient is retrained in the first step, then the OT completes or assists in carrying out the remainder. Once the first step is mastered, the patient goes on to complete the first two steps, then the OT completes or assists with the remainder. This continues until the patient is able to complete all steps independently.

BREAKING AN ACTIVITY INTO SMALLER STEPS: Segmenting brings structure to the activity. This technique reduces the feeling of being overwhelmed and allows the patient to feel a sense of accomplishment without needing to master the entire activity.

DEMONSTRATION: The OT performs the action, task, or activity to illustrate the proper form, correct sequencing, or desired outcome.

HAND OVER HAND: The OT places a hand over the patient to facilitate the desired movement. It should be noted that this technique should only be used when other, less intrusive approaches, such as verbal/visual cueing and/or demonstration, have been deemed ineffective.

REPETITION: New neural pathways, formed in response to novel learning (or retraining), become strengthened with repetition of an action or activity. Over time, the action becomes part of procedural memory and can be performed more accurately and smoothly.

VERBAL/VISUAL CUES: Guiding the patient with words, motions, pictures/signage, notes, etc. to elicit the desired action.

FADING/VANISHING CUES: The amount of information or cues given to produce the correct action is reduced over time. For example, the OT may start with hand-over-hand instruction to facilitate a self-feeding activity, then reduce to verbal cueing, and eventually remove all cues so that the patient completes the activity independently.

ERRORLESS LEARNING: The use of multimodal cues to prevent any mistakes from occurring when relearning a task.

COMPENSATORY COGNTIVIE STRATEGIES: Use of external memory aids, devices, or techniques such as rehearsal or visual imagery.

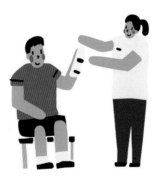

34

PNF Patterns

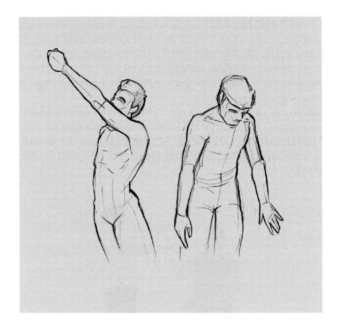

PROPRIOCEPTIVE NEUROMUSCULAR FACILITATION (PNF) PATTERNS

UPPER EXTREMITY DIAGONAL 1 (D1) FLEXION PATTERN:

- Scapula elevation, abduction, upward rotation
- Shoulder flexion, adduction, external rotation
- Elbow flexion or extension
- Forearm supination
- Wrist flexion with radial deviation
- Finger flexion
- Thumb in adduction

UPPER EXTREMITY DIAGONAL 1 (D1) EXTENSION PATTERN:

- Scapula depression, adduction, downward rotation
- Shoulder extension, abduction, internal rotation
- Elbow flexion or extension
- Forearm pronation
- Wrist extension with ulnar deviation
- Finger extension and abduction
- Thumb in palmar abduction

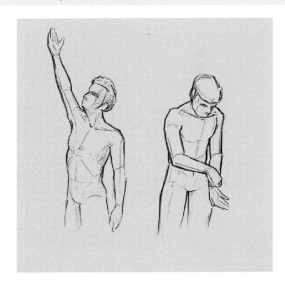

UPPER EXTREMITY DIAGONAL 2 (D2) FLEXION PATTERN:

- Scapula elevation, adduction, upward rotation
- Shoulder flexion, abduction, external rotation
- Elbow in flexion or extension
- Forearm supination
- Wrist extension with radial deviation
- Finger extension and abduction
- Thumb extension

UPPER EXTREMITY DIAGONAL 2 (D2) EXTENSION PATTERN:

- Scapula depression, abduction, downward rotation
- Shoulder extension, adduction, internal rotation
- Elbow flexion or extension
- Forearm pronation
- Wrist flexion with ulnar deviation
- Finger flexion and adduction
- Thumb opposition

35

Adaptive Equipment

ADAPTIVE EQUIPMENT

FEEDING

- Built-up handles
- Lightweight or weighted utensils
- Curved/offset utensils
- Rocker knife
- Scoop plate
- Plate guard
- Swivel spoon
- Nosey cup
- Plates/bowls with suction pad
- U-cuff
- Liftware
- Readi Steadi Anti-Tremor Glove

BATHING

- Shower chair
- Anchored grab bars
- Handheld shower head
- Suction cup handheld shower head holder
- Nonskid mat inside shower
- Rubber-backed mat outside of shower
- Silicone hair scrubber
- No-rinse shampoo cap
- Foot scrubbing pad
- Long-handled sponge/lotion applicator
- Hair funnel for upright bathing
  - **SHOWER/TUB TRANSFER:** Tub transfer bench, sliding transfer bench, anchored grab bars, transfer pole, rolling shower chair, bath lift chair. If patient has tub with sliding glass doors, these can typically be removed and replaced with rod and curtain. If feasible, replace tub with walk-in shower.

DRESSING

- Dressing stick
- Long- or short-handled reacher
- Sock aid
- Compression stocking donner
- Long-handled shoehorn
- Foot funnel
- Button hook
- Magnetic button adaptors
- Zipper pull rings
- No tie/elastic laces
- Velcro clothing
- Clip and pull dressing aid
- A transfer pole can be utilized to stand for pulling pants up over hips

TOILETING

- Bidet
- Handheld bidet sprayer
- Long-handled wiping aid
- **TOILET TRANSFER:** Riser, bedside commode, safety frame, electrical toilet lift, grab bars, stand-alone toilet safety rail, flip-up grab bar, transfer pole, slide board, sit to stand lift, transfer pivot disc.

HYGIENE AND GROOMING

- Electronic toothbrush
- Floss aid
- Suction brush (for hands and under nails)
- Suction denture brush
- U-cuff for holding implements
- Long-handled razor
- Self-inspection mirror
- Long-handled lotion applicator
- Lightweight or weighted long-handled hair brush
- Long-handled swivel head nail clippers

OTHER TRANSFERS

- **CHAIR:** Walker, transfer pivot disc, break extension (for wheelchairs)

- **BED:** Bed ladder, leg lifter, side assist rail, trapeze, low profile box spring if bed is too high
- **COUCH:** Couch risers, couch cane
- **CAR:** Car cane, swivel seat

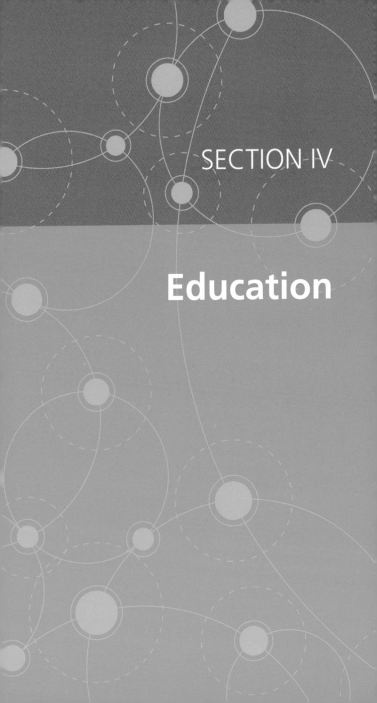

SECTION IV

Education

36

Energy Conservation Techniques

ENERGY CONSERVATION TECHNIQUES: GENERAL

THE 4 'P'S OF ENERGY CONSERVATION:

- **Plan:** Space taxing activity throughout the day and week. Schedule rest breaks during the day. Alternate seated and standing activity. Avoid engaging in activity during hottest time of the day (especially when temperature exceeds 80°F).
- **Prioritize:** Schedule the day considering highest-priority tasks as well as peak energy times.
- **Pace:** Balance rest and activity. Do not rush through tasks. Rest **prior** to feeling tired in order to proactively avoid fatigue.
- **Positioning and proper body mechanics**: See Education: Proper Body Mechanics

DECREASE SHORTNESS OF BREATH

- Utilize effective **breathing patterns**:
  - Pursed-lip breathing
  - Diaphragmatic breathing
- **Use good posture** in order for diaphragm to flatten, producing expansion of thoracic cavity and lungs.
- **Synchronize breath and movement** in accordance with intra-abdominal pressure:
  - Inhale during lighter portion of task or with chest expansion such as reaching up to put dishes in cupboard or overhead to don shirt.
  - Exhale during strenuous portion of task such as when lifting objects or when reducing space in the abdominal and chest cavities, e.g., reaching down to tie shoes.

OTHER CONSIDERATIONS

- Limit visitors during times of recovery.
- Ask for help when the demand of the task exceeds ability.

ENERGY CONSERVATION TECHNIQUES: ACTIVITY OF DAILY LIVING (ADL) SPECIFIC

BATHING

- **Sit during showers** and lean forward while supporting forearms on legs (**tripod posture**) to wash hair. Keeping head and arms lowered and supported decreases cardiac workload.
- Maintain a **well-ventilated space** and keep temperature of water slightly lowered to reduce steam content for easier breathing. If patient wears **oxygen**, ensure it is kept on for the duration of the shower.
- **Utilize adaptive equipment** to decrease need for leaning and reaching. Tools for ease of bathing include shower chair or transfer bench, handheld shower head (with suction cup shower head holder for easy access next to seated patient), and long-handled sponge.
- Don **terry cloth robe** instead of using a towel for drying.

DRESSING

- **Sit for all dressing activity.** Use a chair with armrests for ease of sit <> stand transfers while dressing.
- **Utilize tools** to reduce bending and reaching. These may include dressing stick, reacher, sock aid, and long-handled shoehorn.
- **Don garments together**, e.g., thread underwear and pants over legs and hips together so that only one sit to stand is required.
- **Wear loose-fitting garments with zippers or Velcro**, as they are less fatiguing to don/doff than pullovers.

HYGIENE AND GROOMING

- **Have a chair available** in or near the bathroom for use during hygiene and grooming activities.
- Keep all **frequently used items within reach**.
- **Rest forearms on counter (tripod posture)** while brushing teeth, washing face, shaving, etc.

- **Use electric implements** when possible, such as an electric toothbrush or razor.

TOILETING

- **Utilize adaptive equipment** to reduce exertion, such as a bidet, riser, and grab bars.
- **Use a bedside commode** placed next to bed at night to reduce ambulation distance.
- **Wear pants with elastic waistbands** as opposed to zipper or button closures for ease of pulling up and down.

FEEDING

- Wait until at least **30 min** after eating to engage in activity.

ENERGY CONSERVATION TECHNIQUES: INSTRUMENTAL ACTIVITIES OF DAILY LIVING (IADL) SPECIFIC

MEALS, FOOD PREP, SHOPPING

- **Prepare and cook food in bulk** and freeze or refrigerate portions for later.
- **Keep a bar stool or counter stool nearby** to sit while preparing food.
- Rearrange kitchen items so that the **most frequently used items are at waist or shoulder height** to avoid bending down or reaching.
- **Use power items** such as an electric can opener, jar opener, and food chopper/processor.
- Utilize grocery store food **delivery or curbside pickup**.
- Have meal kits or **prepared meals delivered to doorstep**.
  - If low income, utilize community support programs such as Meals on Wheels.
- **Use motorized carts** for grocery shopping.
- **Organize grocery list** by food isle.

HOUSEKEEPING

- **Create a chore schedule** to spread work out over the week. Clean one room or area per day.
- **Soak dishes** prior to washing.
- **Use cart or wheeled walker** to transport items.
- If possible, consider **robotic vacuum** for cleaning floors.
- **Use a long-handled reacher** to retrieve items off of floor or from high shelves.

(Energy conservation principles and techniques (n.d.).)

EDUCATION

37

Fall Prevention

FALL PREVENTION

HOME MODIFICATIONS

- **Keep clear, open pathways.** Remove any trip hazards.
- **Remove throw rugs** or use double-sided tape to secure properly to floor. Rug pads are beneficial in preventing shifting/slipping of rugs; however, these do not secure edges.
- **Install handrails** on both sides of stairway approximately 36 inches from ground, extending full length of stairs.
- **Install grab bars** next to toilet, at entrance to shower/tub, by stairs leading to front door, garage, or living room that do not have handrail.
- Use appropriate **adaptive equipment/durable medical equipment**.
- **Keep frequently used items within reach** to avoid using stepstool.
- **Use adequate lighting** including nightlights.
- **Install contrast strips/bright-colored tape** on edge of stairs and raised thresholds.

LIFESTYLE/HEALTHY HABITS

- Be consistent with an **exercise program** and include a **balance component**.
- **Eat well and stay hydrated.**
- Ensure **sufficient vitamin D, calcium and magnesium** intake for bone health.
- Schedule **annual checkups** and eye exams.
  - Include a bone density check.
- Be aware of any **side effects** of medications.
- Use an **ambulation device** if advised.
- **Pause when transitioning** between lying, sitting, and standing to avoid lightheadedness.

- **Avoid flip-flop style footwear.** Shoes and slippers should be properly fitting, closed-toe and heel, with rubber soles.

BE PREPARED THE EVENT OF A FALL

- Wear a **call button, medical alert device**, or keep cell phone nearby.
- **Simulate a fall scenario:** Practice self-assessing for injury, summoning assistance in the event of an injury, or fall recovery procedure if uninjured.

(Fall prevention resources One Step Ahead Fall Prevention Program (n.d.).)

EDUCATION

38

Joint Protection Principles

JOINT PROTECTION PRINCIPLES

- **Engage in a strengthening and range-of-motion (ROM) program** to maintain joint integrity. Work in a pain-free range to prevent intra-articular pressure.
- **Avoid keeping a joint in the same position** for long periods.
- **Use the largest/strongest joints when possible,** such as pushing up on armrests with a flat hand (weight is primarily absorbed through wrist joint) rather than pushing up using knuckles; or using legs rather than spine to lift heavy objects.
- **Distribute weight evenly.** This might include wearing a backpack instead of a purse or holding an object with both hands.
- **Avoid rotational forces** such as twisting.
- **Find balance** between rest and movement. Stop activities **before** the joint becomes painful.
- **Explore orthoses** such as braces or splints to support weak joints and reduce strain.
- **Use proper body mechanics.** See Education: Proper Body Mechanics.
- **Practice good posture.** When using a walker, forward-flexed posture can cause increased weight bearing through the joints of the shoulders, wrists, and hands. Educate in proper postural alignment in order to redistribute weight through the lower extremities.
- **Utilize adaptive equipment** to perform activities of daily living/instrumental activities of daily living (ADLs/IADLs), e.g.:
  - **Feeding:** Built-up handles or lightweight utensils, rocker, or angled knife to cut food.
  - **Dressing:** Velcro closure, dressing stick, sock aid, long-handled shoehorn, reacher, zipper pull, elastic shoelaces.

- **Bathing:** Shower chair/transfer bench, grab bars, long-handled sponge, handheld shower head.
- **Toileting:** Bidet, grab bars, long-handled personal hygiene aid, raised toilet seat.
- **Hygiene and grooming:** Electric tools or implements with built-up handles or long handles, floss aid.
- **IADLs:** Door lever handles, built-up writing utensils, electric can and jar opener, food processor, knob turner on stove, rubber grips on faucets, reacher, two-handled pots and pans, gardening kneeler.
- **Mobility-related equipment:** An upright walker or a platform attached to a front wheel walker (FWW) can be used to distribute weight through the forearms as opposed to a regular walker that places weight through the wrists and hands. A luggage roller or walker with tray can be utilized to transport loads.

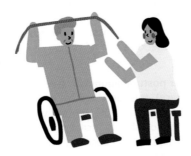

EDUCATION

39

Proper Body Mechanics

PROPER BODY MECHANICS

Static posture:
- **Proper postural alignment**:
  - **Line of gravity** should pass through lobe of ear, shoulder joint, hip joint, anterior to midline of knee, anterior to lateral malleolus with symmetry of shoulders and pelvis.
  - The **spine should be in a neutral position** with normal curvature of the cervical, thoracic, and lumbar regions.
  - Once proper postural alignment has been established, encourage patients to **assess their posture throughout the day** by checking in a mirror.

Dynamic posture:
- Ensure **proper postural alignment** (see above).
- **Stabilize (brace) this position** by engaging muscles of abdomen with at least 20% tension with all movement. Abdominal tension should increase to meet the demands of the movement. In this position, compression forces are distributed away from intervertebral discs.
- Maintain good posture with a **stabilized core and neutral spine and pelvis** during activity.
- Hinge forward at the **hips** instead of curving the spine.
- **Avoid twisting of joints**. For example, avoid using hands to twist open the lid of a jar or to turn the handle of a manual can opener, instead utilize electric devices.

Lifting methods:
- **The squat**: Bend with knees, recruiting muscles of the legs instead of the back.
- **Diagonal lift**: Place one foot in front of the other in a staggered stance around the object, lift with leg muscles.

- **Half kneel lift:** For lifting lighter objects, step forward, bending the front knee while bending the back knee down to kneel on the ground, lift with leg muscles.
- **Golfer's lift:** Hinge forward at the hips while lifting one leg straight behind and maintaining a straight spine.

Lifting techniques:
- **Bring load close to body:** Do not push, pull, or lift when load is outside of base of support. Engage core and exhale while lifting.
- **Use proper lifting techniques:** Always tighten abdominal muscles and exhale during lift portion.
- **Avoid torsional loading and compression-tension forces.** For example, face the object prior to lifting and turn with the whole body.
- **Keep load close to body** for transport.
- **Set up workspace height** to avoid poor posture.

Ease stress on spine:
- When standing for long periods (such as while washing dishes), **lift one foot and place it on a low stool** or the inside of a low cabinet.
- **Change positions frequently.**

EDUCATION

40

Surgical Precautions: Cardiac

SURGICAL PRECAUTIONS

CARDIAC

STERNAL PRECAUTIONS FOR OPEN HEART SURGERY

- **No lifting** >5–8 lbs.
- **No pushing or pulling** with upper extremities.
- **No internal rotation with extension** (reaching behind back) or bilateral abduction.
- **No bilateral shoulder flexion** above 90°.
- **Perform log roll** into and out of bed.
- **Avoid twisting** of trunk.
- With gentle pressure, **hold pillow over heart to act as a splint** during a cough or sneeze.
- **Do not use upper extremities to push up** from sitting or to reach back and lower into sitting.
- **Minimize pressure placed on walker** through upper extremities.

All sternal precautions are generally observed for 6–8 weeks

PACEMAKER PRECAUTIONS

- The involved upper extremity may be in a **sling for the first 24 h** postoperatively.
- **No lifting** >5 lbs.
- **No shoulder flexion or abduction** >90° (light activity with the involved upper extremity is allowed).

- **Minimize pressure placed on walker** through involved upper extremity.

All pacemaker precautions are generally observed for 4–6 weeks

ANGIOPLASTY, STENT, AND CARDIAC CATHETERIZATION

- **No lifting** >10 lbs for 1 week.
- **Avoid strenuous activity** for 1 month.

ONGOING PACEMAKER CONTRAINDICATIONS

- Use of electrical stimulation (**e-stim**).
- Use of transcutaneous electrical nerve stimulation (**TENS unit**).

These are general guidelines only and are not intended to serve as protocols for postoperative care. Clinicians should follow precautions and protocols as set forth by the referring surgeon and the facility in which the patient is being treated.

41

Surgical Precautions: Orthopedic

SURGICAL PRECAUTIONS

ORTHOPEDIC

SPINAL (LAMINECTOMY/DECOMPRESSION/DISCECTOMY)

- **No bending forward >90°** or raising knees above hips.
- **No pushing, pulling, or lifting >5 lbs.**
- **No twisting** (turn with whole body rather than spine).
- **Perform log roll** into and out of bed.
- **Keep spine in a neutral position** throughout the day.

TOTAL KNEE ARTHROPLASTY/TKA

- **No rolled-up towel** or pillow behind knee.
- **No kneeling.**
- **Do not torque/twist knee.**

TOTAL HIP ARTHROPLASTY/THA

- POSTERIOR APPROACH
  - **No hip flexion >90°.**
  - **No adduction** beyond midline.
  - **No internal rotation.**
- ANTERIOR APPROACH
  - **No hip extension.**
  - **No abduction.**
  - **No adduction** beyond midline.
  - **No external rotation.**

All precautions are generally observed for 6–8 weeks.

FEMUR OPEN REDUCTION INTERNAL FIXATION/ORIF/PINNING

- Typically, patients are **non-weight bearing, toe-touch, or partial weight bearing** for first 6–8 weeks and progress to full weight bearing pending individual progress.

TOTAL SHOULDER REPLACEMENT/HEMIARTHROPLASTY/TSA

- **Sling should be worn continuously for 3–4 weeks** unless bathing, dressing, or performing active range of motion (AROM) below shoulder.

- **No AROM of shoulder;** however, **AROM below shoulder (elbow, wrist, and hand) is important** to avoid stiffness/contractures.

- **Avoid internal rotation and adduction together with extension,** which occur when reaching behind back for bathroom hygiene or to tuck in shirt.

- **No lifting, pushing, or pulling.**

- Do not use upper extremities to **push up from sitting or to reach back and lower** into sitting.

JOINT PROTECTION OF REVERSE TOTAL SHOULDER REPLACEMENT/R-TSA

The same precautions as a conventional total shoulder apply; however, there is a higher occurrence of joint dislocation following reverse total shoulder, with the most provoking combination being in the above-mentioned position of internal rotation and adduction together with extension. As such, it is imperative that patients are educated in **compensatory techniques for all activities of daily living (ADLs) that require reaching behind the back.** Additionally, passive range of motion (PROM) into shoulder internal rotation is generally avoided until 6 weeks post op.

NONOPERATIVE PROXIMAL HUMERAL FRACTURE AND PROXIMAL HUMERAL FRACTURE OPEN REDUCTION INTERNAL FIXATION/ORIF

- **Sling should be worn continuously for 3–6 weeks,** unless bathing, dressing, or performing exercises.

- **No AROM of shoulder;** however, **AROM below shoulder (elbow, wrist, and hand) is important** to avoid stiffness/contractures.

EDUCATION

- **No lifting, pushing, or pulling.**
- Do not use upper extremities to **push up from sitting or to reach back and lower** into sitting.

ROTATOR CUFF REPAIR SURGERY

- **Sling should be worn continuously for 6 weeks** unless bathing or performing AROM below shoulder.
- **No AROM of shoulder;** however, **AROM below shoulder (elbow, wrist, and hand) is important** to avoid stiffness or contractures.
- **No lifting, pushing, or pulling.**
- **Take caution with shoulder motion behind back.**
- Do not use upper extremities to **push up from sitting or to reach back and lower** into sitting.

These are general guidelines only and are not intended to serve as protocols for postoperative care. Clinicians should follow precautions and protocols as set forth by the referring surgeon and the facility in which the patient is being treated.

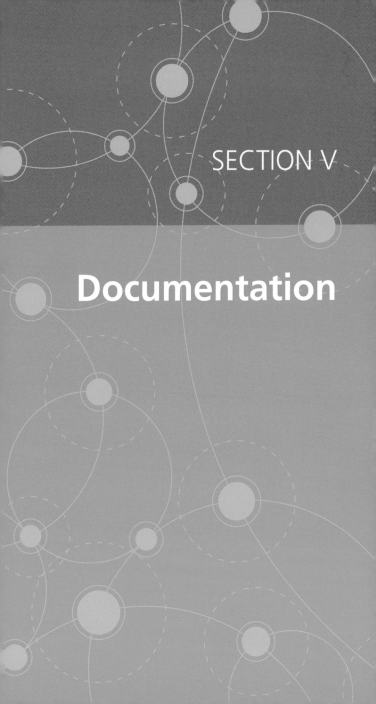

SECTION V

Documentation

42

Reason for Referral Narrative

HOSPITAL SETTING:

Mr/Mrs (name) is a(n) (age)-year-old (female/male) admitted to (hospital) for (diagnosis) in the setting of (any pertinent/chronic disorders in health history). The patient's current presentation demonstrates a significant change in condition and ability in various areas including (activities of daily living [ADLs], instrumental activities of daily living [IADLs], mobility-related ADLs [MR-ADLs], functional transfers, fine motor/gross motor coordination, activity tolerance, sitting/standing balance, proprioception, sensation, safety/judgment, and cognition). S/he exhibits (fair/good/excellent) potential to improve with skilled occupational therapy treatment in order to (meet all goals/return to Prior level of function [PLOF]/safely Discharge [DC] to home setting).

SKILLED NURSING FACILITY:

Mr/Mrs (name) is a(n) (age)-year-old (female/male) admitted to (skilled nursing facility) following a (#)-day qualifying stay in (hospital) due to (diagnosis) in the setting of (any pertinent/chronic disorders in health history). Patient progressed as expected in hospital, or hospital stay was complicated by (any issues that occurred). The patient's current presentation demonstrates a significant change in condition and ability in various areas including (activities of daily living [ADLs], instrumental activities of daily living [IADLs], mobility-related ADLs [MR-ADLs], functional transfers, fine motor/gross motor coordination, activity tolerance, sitting/standing balance, proprioception, sensation, safety/judgment, and cognition). S/he exhibits (fair/good/excellent) potential to improve with skilled occupational therapy treatment in order to (meet all goals/return to PLOF/safely DC to home setting).

DOCUMENTATION

HOME HEALTH SETTING:

Mr/Mrs (name) is a(n) (age)-year-old (female/male admitted to (home health agency) following a stay in (hospital) due to (diagnosis) in the setting of (any pertinent/chronic disorders in health history). Patient was subsequently transferred to (skilled nursing facility [SNF]) for further recovery and stabilization prior to discharge home. During hospital/SNF course, patient progressed as expected, or hospital/SNF stay was complicated by (any issues that occurred). This patient has now returned home and continues to demonstrate below baseline functioning in the areas of (activities of daily living [ADLs], instrumental activities of daily living [IADLs], mobility-related ADLs [MR-ADLs], functional transfers, fine motor/gross motor coordination, activity tolerance, sitting/standing balance, proprioception, sensation, safety/judgment, and cognition). S/he exhibits (fair/good/excellent) potential to improve with skilled occupational therapy treatment in order to (meet all goals/return to PLOF).

43

SOAP Note/Treatment Encounter Note

SOAP NOTE/TREATMENT ENCOUNTER NOTE

SUBJECTIVE

Captures the subjective experience of the patient:

- New information since the most recent visit pertaining to health status or changes in condition, such as any lifted precautions or new symptoms.
- Complaints of pain, fatigue, or other symptoms experienced before, during, or after therapy.
- A direct quote that exemplifies the patient's perception of progress or attitude regarding recovery.
- Applicable questions, concerns, or desires.
- Pertinent information reported by caregivers.

Example: An 82-year-old F, s/p R cerebral vascular accident (CVA) with L-sided hemiplegia and mild unilateral neglect, inpatient rehab setting, 60 min treatment (tx) session.

- Patient reports frustration with lack of coordination and control of left upper extremity (L UE), though continues to experience improvements with functional activity: "This arm didn't want to behave but I was able to get my shirt on without help this morning for the first time!" Patient reports 2/10 hemiplegic shoulder pain and states that pain reduction techniques from previous tx session had a beneficial and lasting effect.

OBJECTIVE

Contains quantifiable data as well as details of the treatment intervention:

- Objective measures and observations such as assessment scores, range of motion (ROM), and manual muscle testing (MMT) values.

- Skilled interventions should be documented by clearly indicating the specific areas of impairment or functional limitations that the activity aims to address and improve. Some examples include:

  - Functional strength

  - Functional range of motion

  - Static balance (sitting and standing)

  - Dynamic balance (sitting and standing)

  - Leaning and reaching outside of base of support (BOS)

  - Trunk control

  - Postural alignment

  - Weightbearing (WB)

  - Weight shifting in various directions

  - Bilateral upper extremity (BUE) integration and coordination

  - Shoulder flexion

  - Fine/gross motor control

  - Prehensile/grasp patterns

  - Pain

  - Safety awareness

  - Functional activity tolerance

  - Functional transfers

  - Mobility-related ADL (MR-ADL)

  - Crossing midline

  - Proprioception

  - Neglect

  - Spasticity

- Hyper/hypotonicity
- Cognition
  - Problem solving
  - Safety awareness and judgment
  - Comprehension
  - Attention
  - Sequencing
  - Planning
  - Memory
  - Orientation
- The level and extent of assistance needed during the session, including physical assistance (minimal, moderate, maximum, or total dependence), types of cues provided (verbal, tactile, etc.), and utilization of demonstrations.
- Specific retraining techniques such as forward/backward chaining, errorless learning, or vanishing cues.
- Grading strategies implemented to ensure a "just right" challenge such as increasing/decreasing the complexity of a task, using repitition, or segmenting a task.
- Recommendations of task modifications, environmental modifications, or adaptive equipment.
- How the patient responded during and after the activity.

Example continued from above: Occupational therapist (OT) performed scapulothoracic mobilizations of affected L UE with patient in side lying consisting of gliding, rotations, and distraction. Decreased soft tissue restriction noted with upward rotation. Hot pack placed on L shoulder during weight-bearing activity to decrease hemiplegic shoulder pain; patient sat on mat leaning laterally on open hand to bear weight through extremity to provide proprioceptive input and improve proximal joint stability. Min A to maintain position with tapping technique performed over triceps for 5×30 seconds. Patient participated in therapeutic activity to promote proprioceptive neuromuscular facilitation (PNF) patterns, fine motor (FM) coordination, and crossing midline: Patient reached down to retrieve puzzle piece from low surface using extension patterns (box placed to right then left of patient in order to facilitate both D1/D2 patterns). Visual scanning of box from left to right to find edge pieces with hand-over-hand facilitation of pincer grasp for retrieval. Initially, patient had difficulty finding pieces, thus OT guided pt in organized search pattern, ensuring visual tracking to left side. Max A to complete D1/D2 flexion patterns in order to place each piece on high surface and release grasp. Review of hemiplegic dressing techniques to don shirt, performed with set up, stand by assist (SBA), no verbal cues needed.

L shoulder: active range of motion (AROM) 45°/passive range of motion (PROM) 120°

ASSESSMENT

Summarizes the OT's interpretation of the data from the previous two sections (subjective and objective) in order to create a narrative regarding the patient's current status and trajectory toward meeting goals:

- Using clinical reasoning, determine if/how patient is progressing toward goals, including functional levels and carryover of technique/information.

- Justify treatment based on patient's response to skilled interventions.

- Document progress made since last tx session and during the current session.

- State how level of motivation and participation affect progress.

- If patient is making limited progress or has plateaued with therapy:

  - What barriers exist to reaching goals?

  - What changes should be made to treatment interventions?

Example continued from above: Patient's frustration with limited use of L UE indicates improved directed attention toward left side. Increased awareness is also evidenced by recent spontaneous use of L UE to engage in self-care tasks. An 8° increase in AROM of L shoulder allows patient to participate in functional reach activities, albeit in a limited capacity. Pain continues to be well managed, allowing for maximum participation with treatment. Patient demonstrates good carryover of hemiplegic dressing techniques; progress toward meeting self-care goals and a strong desire to return to her previous living situation indicate good potential to return to her prior level of function.

PLAN

Outlines what the OT intends to do going forward based on data from the previous three sections:

- Focus of the next treatment session including the targeted impairments, occupations, or specific interventions.
- Details of any information the OT would like to follow up on (e.g., communication with interdisciplinary team [IDT], caregivers, referrals, etc.).
- Changes to the treatment plan.
- Ensure that documentation could help other clinicians understand the focus of future visits.

Example continued from above: Patient would benefit from skilled instruction in lower body dressing and stand pivot transfer wheelchair (WC) <> toilet at next visit. Plan to administer modified Barthel index at next visit. Continue with pain reduction strategy at each visit, including scapular mobilizations (scap mobs), positioning techniques, and use of thermal agents.

44

Homebound Status

HOMEBOUND STATUS

A patient must be homebound in order to qualify for home health services. According to Medicare guidelines, leaving the home must require a considerable and taxing effort due to injury, illness, the need for help (from another person or mobility device), or the patient must have a condition that makes leaving the home contraindicated ("6.2.1.1 – Certification Requirements," 2017). The following are specific examples that can be used in documentation to demonstrate that a patient is homebound:

- Fatigue/weakness
- Fall with injury
- Immunocompromised
- Shortness of breath (SOB) with minimal exertion
- Requires frequent rest breaks
- Unable to toilet in public
- High pain levels
- Use of narcotic pain meds causing disorientation, drowsiness, or dizziness
- Cardiopulmonary disease exacerbation (risk of desaturation)
- Unable to walk community distances
- Requires supportive devices such as electric wheelchair and special transport
- Non-weight-bearing
- Status post (S/p) surgery
- Surgical wound: risk of infection or delayed healing
- Requires an attendant due to:
  - Impaired cognition (not able to safely enter/negotiate community)
  - Wandering/exit-seeking behavior
  - Unsafe gait pattern
  - Poor balance

- Inability to transfer self
  - Patients are allowed to attend, without risk of losing homebound status, medical appointments, adult day care center, or special events such as a family reunion, funeral, graduation, or religious services. Patients are also allowed occasional visits to the barber or hair salon. (The homebound requirement.)

45

Skilled Terminology

- Achieved
- Adapted
- Adjusted
- Administered
- Advanced
- Advised
- Analyzed
- Assessed
- Clarified
- Collaborated
- Communicated
- Consulted
- Corrected
- Demonstrated
- Directed
- Educated
- Enabled
- Endorsed
- Engaged
- Established
- Facilitated
- Identified
- Implemented
- Improved
- Increased
- Instructed
- Integrated
- Measured
- Modified
- Observed
- Prioritized
- Progressed
- Promoted
- Provided
- Reduced
- Restored
- Retrained
- Simplified
- Simulated
- Stabilized
- Structured
- Targeted

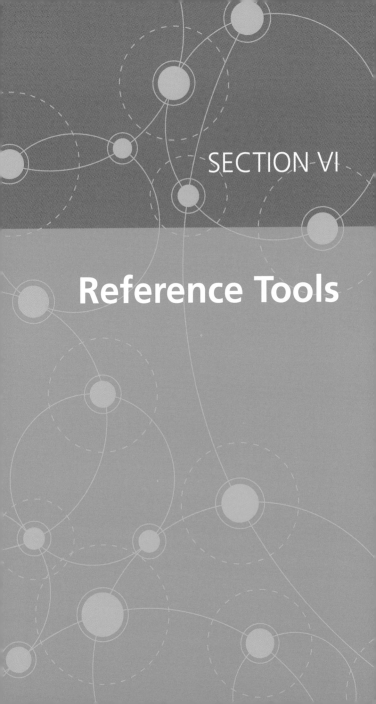

SECTION VI

Reference Tools

Anatomical Planes and Orientation

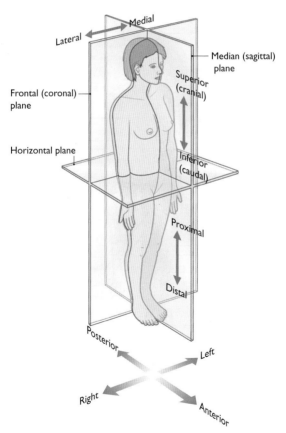

Anatomical planes and orientation

Muscle Diagrams

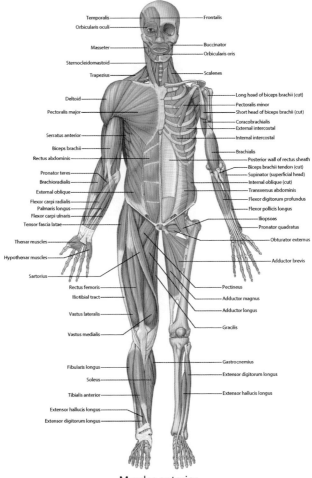

Muscles anterior

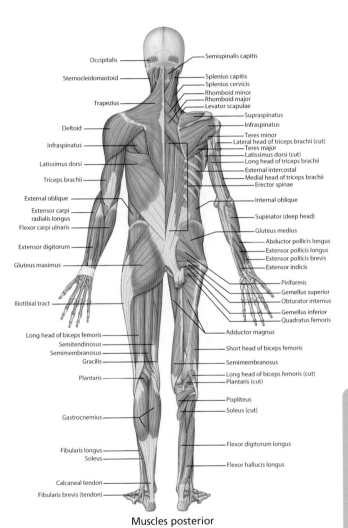

Occipitalis — Semispinalis capitis
Sternocleidomastoid — Splenius capitis
Splenius cervicis
Rhomboid minor
Rhomboid major
Trapezius — Levator scapulae
Supraspinatus
Infraspinatus
Deltoid — Teres minor
Lateral head of triceps brachii (cut)
Infraspinatus — Teres major
Latissimus dorsi (cut)
Long head of triceps brachii
Latissimus dorsi — External intercostal
Medial head of triceps brachii
Triceps brachii — Erector spinae
External oblique — Internal oblique
Extensor carpi
radialis longus — Supinator (deep head)
Flexor carpi ulnaris — Gluteus medius
Extensor digitorum — Abductor pollicis longus
Extensor pollicis longus
Extensor pollicis brevis
Gluteus maximus — Extensor indicis
Piriformis
Gemellus superior
Obturator internus
Iliotibial tract — Gemellus inferior
Quadratus femoris
Long head of biceps femoris — Adductor magnus
Semitendinosus
Semimembranosus — Short head of biceps femoris
Gracilis — Semimembranosus
Long head of biceps femoris (cut)
Plantaris — Plantaris (cut)
Popliteus
Soleus (cut)
Gastrocnemius —
Fibularis longus — Flexor digitorum longus
Soleus — Flexor hallucis longus
Calcaneal tendon —
Fibularis brevis (tendon) —

Muscles posterior

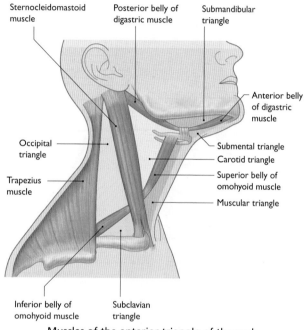

Muscles of the anterior triangle of the neck

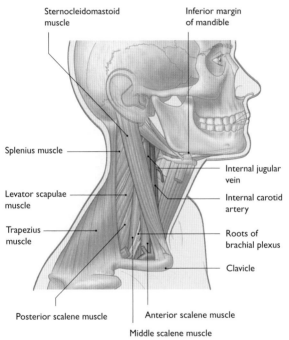

Deep muscles of the neck and posterior triangle of the neck

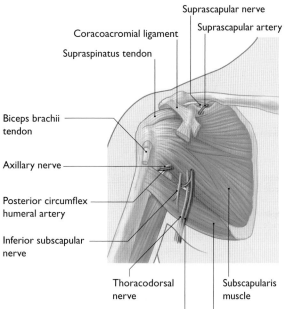

Scapular muscles (right, anterior aspect)

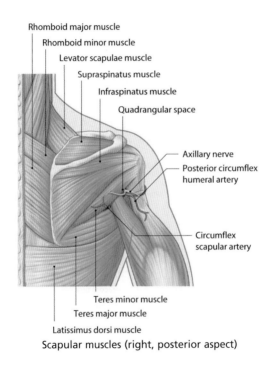

Rhomboid major muscle
Rhomboid minor muscle
Levator scapulae muscle
Supraspinatus muscle
Infraspinatus muscle
Quadrangular space

Axillary nerve
Posterior circumflex humeral artery

Circumflex scapular artery

Teres minor muscle
Teres major muscle
Latissimus dorsi muscle
Scapular muscles (right, posterior aspect)

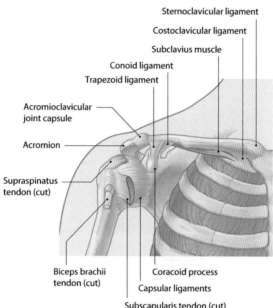

Glenohumeral joint (right, anterior aspect)

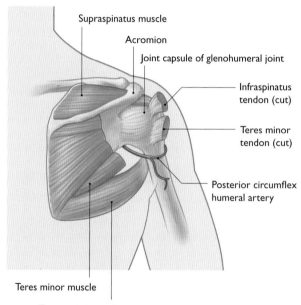

Supraspinatus muscle

Acromion

Joint capsule of glenohumeral joint

Infraspinatus tendon (cut)

Teres minor tendon (cut)

Posterior circumflex humeral artery

Teres minor muscle

Teres major muscle

Glenohumeral joint (right, posterior aspect)

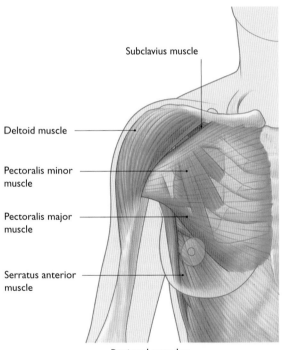

Subclavius muscle

Deltoid muscle

Pectoralis minor
muscle

Pectoralis major
muscle

Serratus anterior
muscle

Pectoral muscles

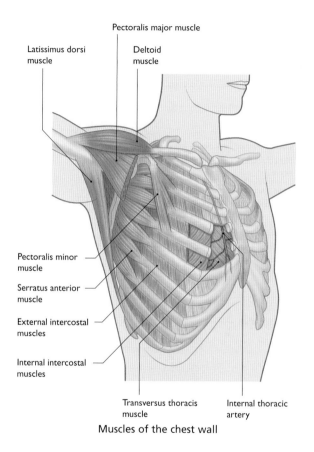

Muscles of the chest wall

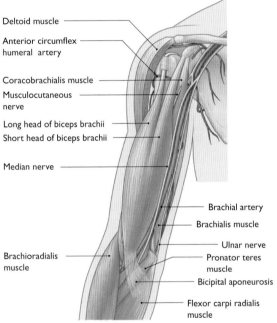

Deltoid muscle

Anterior circumflex humeral artery

Coracobrachialis muscle

Musculocutaneous nerve

Long head of biceps brachii

Short head of biceps brachii

Median nerve

Brachial artery

Brachialis muscle

Ulnar nerve

Pronator teres muscle

Bicipital aponeurosis

Brachioradialis muscle

Flexor carpi radialis muscle

Upper extremity (right, anterior aspect)

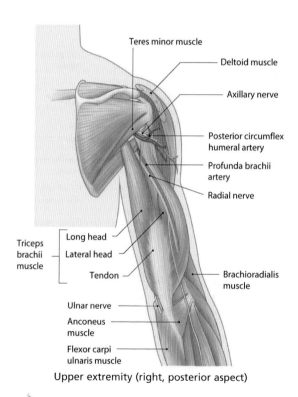

Upper extremity (right, posterior aspect)

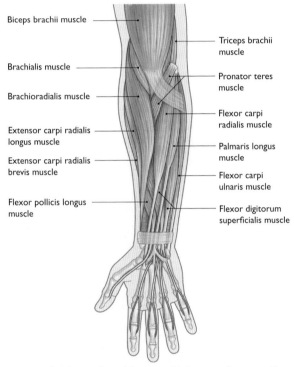

Biceps brachii muscle

Triceps brachii muscle

Brachialis muscle

Pronator teres muscle

Brachioradialis muscle

Flexor carpi radialis muscle

Extensor carpi radialis longus muscle

Palmaris longus muscle

Extensor carpi radialis brevis muscle

Flexor carpi ulnaris muscle

Flexor pollicis longus muscle

Flexor digitorum superficialis muscle

Superficial muscles of forearm (right, anterior aspect)

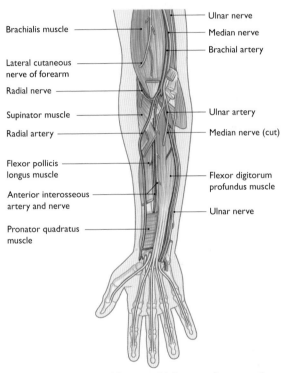

Brachialis muscle

Lateral cutaneous
nerve of forearm

Radial nerve

Supinator muscle

Radial artery

Flexor pollicis
longus muscle

Anterior interosseous
artery and nerve

Pronator quadratus
muscle

Ulnar nerve

Median nerve

Brachial artery

Ulnar artery

Median nerve (cut)

Flexor digitorum
profundus muscle

Ulnar nerve

Deep structures of forearm (right, anterior aspect)

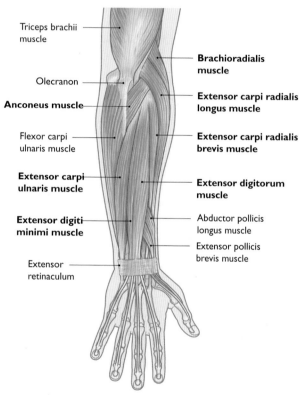

Triceps brachii muscle

Olecranon

Anconeus muscle

Flexor carpi ulnaris muscle

Extensor carpi ulnaris muscle

Extensor digiti minimi muscle

Extensor retinaculum

Brachioradialis muscle

Extensor carpi radialis longus muscle

Extensor carpi radialis brevis muscle

Extensor digitorum muscle

Abductor pollicis longus muscle

Extensor pollicis brevis muscle

Superficial muscles of forearm (right, posterior aspect)

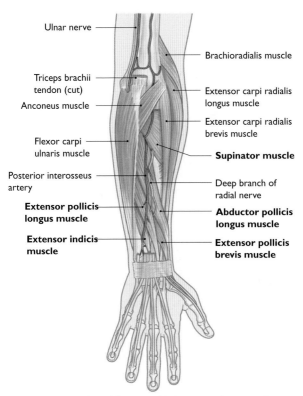

Ulnar nerve

Triceps brachii tendon (cut)

Anconeus muscle

Flexor carpi ulnaris muscle

Posterior interosseus artery

Extensor pollicis longus muscle

Extensor indicis muscle

Brachioradialis muscle

Extensor carpi radialis longus muscle

Extensor carpi radialis brevis muscle

Supinator muscle

Deep branch of radial nerve

Abductor pollicis longus muscle

Extensor pollicis brevis muscle

Deep muscles of forearm (right, posterior aspect)

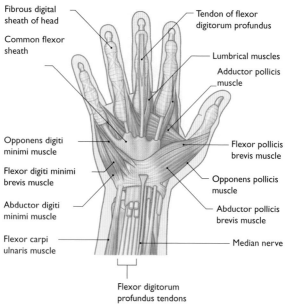

Fibrous digital sheath of head

Common flexor sheath

Opponens digiti minimi muscle

Flexor digiti minimi brevis muscle

Abductor digiti minimi muscle

Flexor carpi ulnaris muscle

Tendon of flexor digitorum profundus

Lumbrical muscles

Adductor pollicis muscle

Flexor pollicis brevis muscle

Opponens pollicis muscle

Abductor pollicis brevis muscle

Median nerve

Flexor digitorum profundus tendons

Muscles of the anterior (palmar) surface of the hand

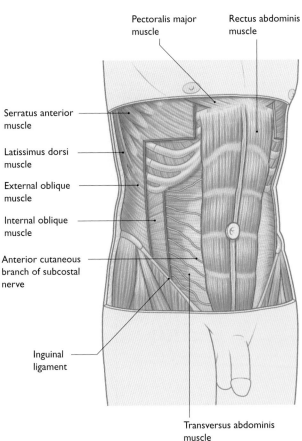

Anterior abdominal wall muscles

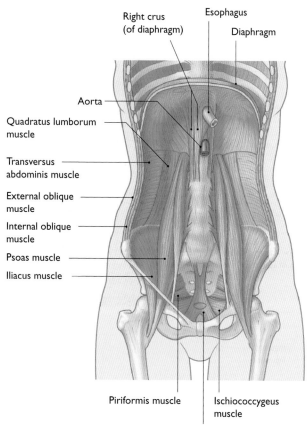

Posterior abdominal wall muscles

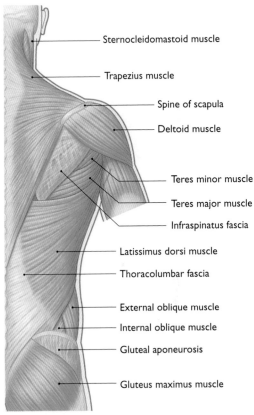

Superficial muscles of the back

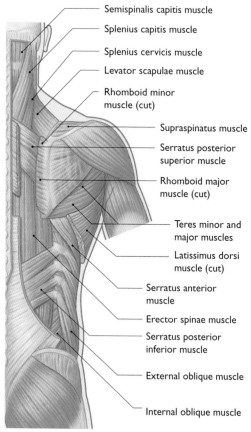

- Semispinalis capitis muscle
- Splenius capitis muscle
- Splenius cervicis muscle
- Levator scapulae muscle
- Rhomboid minor muscle (cut)
- Supraspinatus muscle
- Serratus posterior superior muscle
- Rhomboid major muscle (cut)
- Teres minor and major muscles
- Latissimus dorsi muscle (cut)
- Serratus anterior muscle
- Erector spinae muscle
- Serratus posterior inferior muscle
- External oblique muscle
- Internal oblique muscle

Intermediate layer of muscles of the back

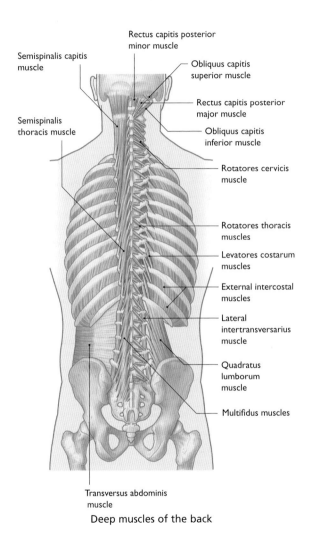

Rectus capitis posterior minor muscle

Semispinalis capitis muscle

Obliquus capitis superior muscle

Rectus capitis posterior major muscle

Semispinalis thoracis muscle

Obliquus capitis inferior muscle

Rotatores cervicis muscle

Rotatores thoracis muscles

Levatores costarum muscles

External intercostal muscles

Lateral intertransversarius muscle

Quadratus lumborum muscle

Multifidus muscles

Transversus abdominis muscle

Deep muscles of the back

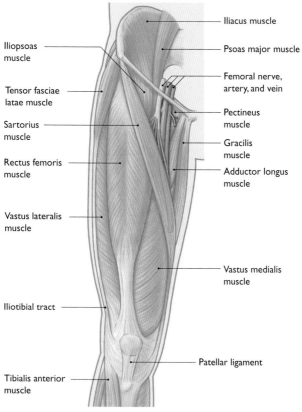

Iliacus muscle

Psoas major muscle

Femoral nerve, artery, and vein

Iliopsoas muscle

Tensor fasciae latae muscle

Sartorius muscle

Rectus femoris muscle

Vastus lateralis muscle

Iliotibial tract

Tibialis anterior muscle

Pectineus muscle

Gracilis muscle

Adductor longus muscle

Vastus medialis muscle

Patellar ligament

Superficial muscles of the thigh (right, anterior aspect)

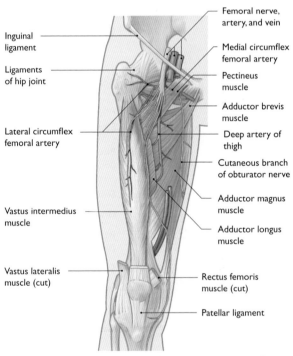

Inguinal ligament

Ligaments of hip joint

Lateral circumflex femoral artery

Vastus intermedius muscle

Vastus lateralis muscle (cut)

Femoral nerve, artery, and vein

Medial circumflex femoral artery

Pectineus muscle

Adductor brevis muscle

Deep artery of thigh

Cutaneous branch of obturator nerve

Adductor magnus muscle

Adductor longus muscle

Rectus femoris muscle (cut)

Patellar ligament

Deep muscles of the thigh (right, anterior aspect)

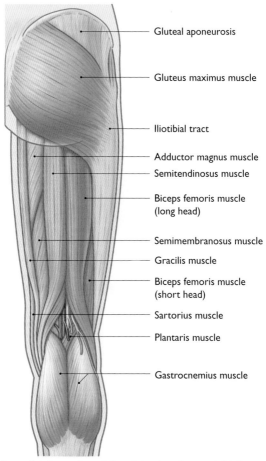

Gluteal aponeurosis

Gluteus maximus muscle

Iliotibial tract

Adductor magnus muscle

Semitendinosus muscle

Biceps femoris muscle
(long head)

Semimembranosus muscle

Gracilis muscle

Biceps femoris muscle
(short head)

Sartorius muscle

Plantaris muscle

Gastrocnemius muscle

Superficial muscles of the gluteal region and thigh
(right, posterior aspect)

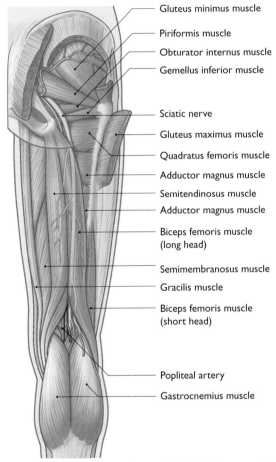

Gluteus minimus muscle

Piriformis muscle

Obturator internus muscle

Gemellus inferior muscle

Sciatic nerve

Gluteus maximus muscle

Quadratus femoris muscle

Adductor magnus muscle

Semitendinosus muscle

Adductor magnus muscle

Biceps femoris muscle
(long head)

Semimembranosus muscle

Gracilis muscle

Biceps femoris muscle
(short head)

Popliteal artery

Gastrocnemius muscle

Deep muscles of the gluteal region and thigh (right, posterior)

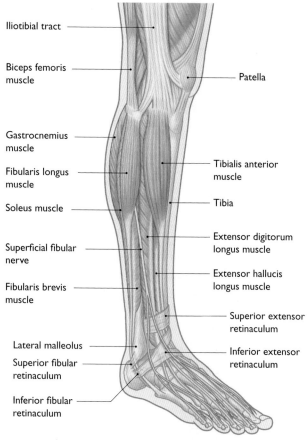

Iliotibial tract

Biceps femoris muscle

Patella

Gastrocnemius muscle

Fibularis longus muscle

Soleus muscle

Superficial fibular nerve

Fibularis brevis muscle

Lateral malleolus

Superior fibular retinaculum

Inferior fibular retinaculum

Tibialis anterior muscle

Tibia

Extensor digitorum longus muscle

Extensor hallucis longus muscle

Superior extensor retinaculum

Inferior extensor retinaculum

Muscles of the anterolateral lower extremity (right)

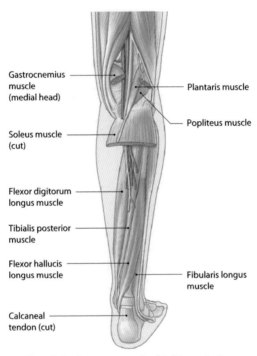

Gastrocnemius muscle (medial head)

Plantaris muscle

Popliteus muscle

Soleus muscle (cut)

Flexor digitorum longus muscle

Tibialis posterior muscle

Flexor hallucis longus muscle

Fibularis longus muscle

Calcaneal tendon (cut)

Deep muscles of the lower extremity (right, posterior aspect)

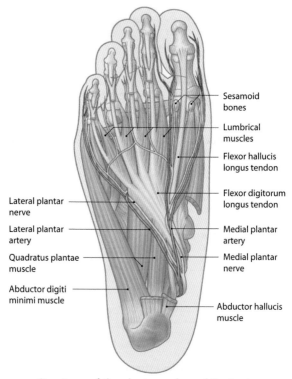

Sesamoid
bones

Lumbrical
muscles

Flexor hallucis
longus tendon

Flexor digitorum
longus tendon

Lateral plantar
nerve

Lateral plantar
artery

Quadratus plantae
muscle

Abductor digiti
minimi muscle

Medial plantar
artery

Medial plantar
nerve

Abductor hallucis
muscle

Structures of the plantar surface of the foot

48

Dermatomes

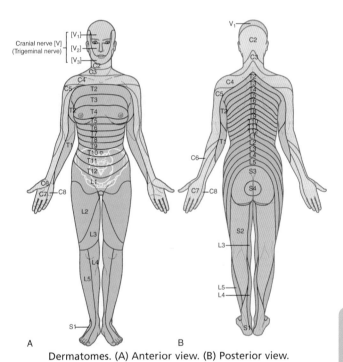

Dermatomes. (A) Anterior view. (B) Posterior view.

49

Lab Values and Implications for Therapy

LAB VALUES AND IMPLICATIONS FOR TX		
COMPLETE BLOOD COUNT (CBC)	NORMAL RANGE	IMPLICATIONS
Hemoglobin (Hgb)	12–16 g/dL (female) 14–17.4 g/dL (male)	>10 g/dL = Regular activity 8–10 g/dL = Light activity, symptoms-based approach **<8 g/dL = Defer therapy**
Hematocrit (HCT)	37%–47% (female) 42%–52% (male)	>25% symptoms-based approach **<25% = Defer therapy** **>60% = Defer therapy**
White blood cells (WBCs)/ leukocytes	5,000–10,000 μL or 5–10 k/μL	> 5,000 μL = Regular activity, take caution if febrile **< 5,000 μL = Defer therapy**
Platelets	140,000–400,000 μL or 140–400 k/μL	>50,000 μL or >50 k/μL = Regular activity 20,000–50,000 μL or 20–50 k/μL = Light activity **<20,000 or <20 k/μL = Defer therapy**

ELECTROLYTE PANEL	NORMAL RANGE	IMPLICATIONS FOR THERAPY
Sodium (Na)	134–142 mEq/L	**Low**/Hyponatremia: Pitting edema, orthostatic hypotension, lethargy, nausea, and vomiting **High**/Hypernatremia: Fluid retention, swelling, impaired cognition, seizure precautions for patients with past medical history, hypertension, tachycardia Symptoms-based approach in determining appropriateness for therapy
Potassium (K)	3.7–5.1 mEq/L	**Low**/Hypokalemia: Weakness, cramps, hypotension, cardiac arrest. **Cardiac risk <2.5 mEq/L** **High**/Hyperkalemia: Weakness/paralysis, bradycardia, ventricular fibrillation, cardiac arrest. **Cardiac risk >5 mEq/L** Symptoms-based approach in determining appropriateness for therapy
Calcium (Ca)	8.6–10.3 mg/dL	**Low**/Hypocalcemia: Impaired cognition, seizures, fatigue, muscle cramps and spasms **High**/Hypercalcemia: Arrhythmia, lethargy, weakness, nausea and vomiting, coma Symptoms-based approach in determining appropriateness for therapy

REFERENCE TOOLS

Magnesium (Mg)	1.2–1.9 mEq/L	**Low**/Hypomagnesemia: Tremors, spasticity, seizures, nystagmus, arrhythmia **High**/Hypermagnesemia: Lethargy, hypotension, weakness, flaccidity, respiratory failure, arrhythmia, paralysis, coma Symptoms-based approach in determining appropriateness for therapy
ENDOCRINE	**NORMAL RANGE**	**IMPLICATIONS FOR THERAPY**
Glucose	70–100 mg/dL	**Low**/Hypoglycemia: **<70 mg/dL** Lethargy, irritability, shaking, extremity weakness, loss of consciousness **High**/Hyperglycemia: **>200 mg/dL** Decreased activity tolerance, extreme fatigue Symptoms-based approach to appropriateness of activity

INTERNATIONAL NORMALIZED RATIO (INR)	**RANGE**
Normal	0.8–1.2
Therapeutic range for stroke prophylaxis	2–2.5
Therapeutic range for venous thromboembolism (VTE) pulmonary embolism (PE) and atrial fibrillation (A-fib)	2–3
Therapeutic range for patients at higher risk such as with prosthetic heart valves	2.5–3.5
Therapeutic range for patients with lupus anticoagulant	3–3.5

INTERNATIONAL NORMALIZED RATIO (INR)	RANGE
Patient at higher risk for bleeding	>3.6
Prothrombin time (PT-INR)	11–13 s (Therapeutic range: 1–2 times normal)
Activated partial thromboplastin time (aPTT)	21–35 s (>70 s signifies risk for spontaneous bleeding)
Therapeutic range for effectiveness of anticoagulant	2–2.5 times normal range (60–109 s)

INR (HIGH)	IMPLICATIONS FOR THERAPY
4.0	Light activity only, symptoms-based approach
5.0	Limited OT eval only, symptoms-based approach
6.0	Defer therapy

CARDIAC ENZYMES	NORMAL	IMPLICATIONS FOR THERAPY
Troponin	<0.034 ng/mL	If patient is diagnosed with myocardial infarction, defer therapy until three consecutive down-trending values.
B-type natriuretic peptide (BNP)	<100 pg/mL	>100–500 Probable heart failure (HF) >500 Indicative of HF Use clinical judgment; likely safe to continue therapy as tolerated as long as patient does not present with: <ul><li>Shortness of breath with minimal activity</li><li>Edema</li><li>Weight gain of >2–3 lb in 24 h</li><li>Chest pain</li></ul>

REFERENCE TOOLS

Lab values current as of 2019 from The American Physical Therapy Association (APTA). The above parameters are general guidelines only and are not meant to take the place of skilled clinical judgment, individual assessment, established protocols, or MD orders.
Academy of Acute Care Physical Therapy (2019).

2020 Alzheimer's disease facts and figures. (2020, March 1). Alzheimer's Association. Retrieved September 6, 2021, from https://alz-journals.onlinelibrary.wiley.com/doi/full/10.1002/alz.12068

Academy of Neurologic Physical Therapy. (n.d.). *Six Minute Walk Test (6MWT)*. Retrieved April 30, 2023, from https://www.neuropt.org/docs/default-source/cpgs/core-outcome-measures/6mwt-pocket-guide-proof9.pdf?sfvrsn=9ee25043_0

6.2.1.1—Certification Requirements. (2017, March 17). [E-book]. In *CMS Manual System* (p. 4). Centers for Medicare & Medicaid Services (CMS).

Academy of Acute Care Physical Therapy. (2019). *Laboratory values interpretation resource*. APA Task Force on Lab Values. https://cdn.ymaws.com/www.aptaacutecare.org/resource/resmgr/docs/2017-Lab-Values-Resource.pdf

Aisen, P.S., Cummings, J., Jack, C.R. et al. On the path to 2025: understanding the Alzheimer's disease continuum. *Alz Res Therapy* 9, 60 (2017). https://doi.org/10.1186/s13195-017-0283-5

Bahmani, D. S., Kesselring, J., Papadimitriou, M., Bansi, J., Pühse, U., Gerber, M., Shaygannejad, V., Holsboer-Trachsler, E., & Brand, S. (2019). In patients with multiple sclerosis, both objective and subjective sleep, depression, fatigue, and paresthesia improved after 3 weeks of regular exercise. *Frontiers in Psychiatry*, 10. https://doi.org/10.3389/fpsyt.2019.00265

Barthel Index. (2020, May 21). *Shirley Ryan AbilityLab*. Retrieved September 5, 2021, from https://www.sralab.org/rehabilitation-measures/barthel-index

Berg Balance Scale. (2020, June 30). *Shirley Ryan AbilityLab*. Retrieved September 5, 2021, from https://www.sralab.org/rehabilitation-measures/berg-balance-scale

Bhattarai, M., & Adhikari, B. (2015). Meaning of life after spinal cord injury. Journal of Chitwan Medical College, 5(2), 12–15.

Bhattarai, M., Smedema, S. M., & Maneewat, K. (2020). An integrative review of factors associated with resilience post-spinal cord injury. *Rehabilitation Counseling Bulletin, 64*(2), 118–127. https://doi.org/10.1177/0034355220938429

Bherer, L., Erickson, K. I., & Liu-Ambrose, T. (2013). A review of the effects of physical activity and exercise on cognitive and brain functions in older adults. *Journal of Aging Research*, 8, 6575083. https://doi.org/10.1155/2013/657508

Bohannon, R. W. (2006). Reference values for the timed up and go test: A descriptive meta-analysis. *PubMed*. Retrieved September 5, 2021, from https://pubmed.ncbi.nlm.nih.gov/16914068/

Canadian Occupational Performance Measure. (2019, June 1). *Shirley Ryan AbilityLab*. Retrieved September 5, 2021, from https://www.sralab.org/rehabilitation-measures/canadian-occupational-performance-measure

Cardiovascular diseases. (2019, June 11). World Health Organization. Retrieved September 8, 2021, from https://www.who.int/health-topics/cardiovascular-diseases#tab=tab_1

Carlsson, A. C., Wändell, P. E., Gigante, B., Leander, K., Hellenius, M. L., & de Faire, U. (2013). Seven modifiable lifestyle factors predict reduced risk for ischemic cardiovascular disease and all-cause mortality regardless of body mass index: A cohort study. *International Journal of Cardiology, 168*(2), 946–952. https://doi.org/10.1016/j.ijcard.2012.10.045

Carrier, S. L., Hicks, A. J., Ponsford, J., & McKay, A. (2021). Managing agitation during early recovery in adults with traumatic brain injury: An international survey. *Annals of Physical and Rehabilitation Medicine, 64*(5), 101532. https://doi.org/10.1016/j.rehab.2021.101532

CDC Prevention Programs. (2018, May). Www.Heart.Org. Retrieved September 8, 2021, from https://www.heart.org/en/get-involved/advocate/federal-priorities/cdc-prevention-programs

Cutts, S. (2007). Cubital tunnel syndrome. *Postgraduate Medical Journal, 83*(975), 28–31. https://doi.org/10.1136/pgmj.2006.047456

Dautel, A. (2019, April 30). Multifactorial intervention for hip and pelvic fracture patients with mild to moderate cognitive impairment: study protocol of a dual-centre randomised controlled trial (OF-CARE). *BMC Geriatrics*. Retrieved September 6, 2021, from https://bmcgeriatr.biomedcentral.com/articles/10.1186/s12877-019-1133-z

Energy Conservation Principles and Techniques. (n.d.). Duke University Department of Physical and Occupational Therapy. Retrieved November 8, 2021, from https://sites.duke.edu/ptot/outpatient-services/patient-resources/energy-conservation

Exercise. (2021). National Multiple Sclerosis Society. Retrieved September 17, 2021, from https://www.nationalmssociety.org/Living-Well-With-MS/Diet-Exercise-Healthy-Behaviors/Exercise

Exercise prescription for patients with multiple sclerosis; potential benefits and practical recommendations. (2017). *PubMed Central (PMC)*. Retrieved September 17, 2021, from https://www.ncbi.nlm.nih.gov/pmc/articles/PMC5602953/

Fall prevention resources One Step Ahead Fall Prevention Program. (n.d.). *Kingcounty.Gov*. Retrieved November 8, 2021, from https://kingcounty.gov/depts/health/emergency-medical-services/community/fall-prevention.aspx

Ferguson, R. J., Palmer, A. J., Taylor, A., Porter, M. L., Malchau, H., & Glyn-Jones, S. (2018). Hip replacement. *The Lancet, 392*(10158), 1662–1671. https://doi.org/10.1016/s0140-6736(18)31777-x

Five Times Sit to Stand Test. (n.d.). Https://Www.Sralab.Org/. https://www.sralab.org/rehabilitation-measures/five-times-sit-to-stand-test

Fletcher, M. (n.d.). *Know the Signs of Stroke—BE FAST*. Duke Health. Retrieved October 22, 1021, from https://www.dukehealth.org/blog/know-signs-of-stroke-be-fast

Functional Independence Measure (FIM). (n.d.). *Physiopedia*. Retrieved September 5, 2021, from https://www.physio-pedia.com/Functional_Independence_Measure_(FIM)

Functional Reach Test/Modified Functional Reach Test. (2013, December 4). *Shirley Ryan AbilityLab*. Retrieved September 5, 2021, from https://www.sralab.org/rehabilitation-measures/functional-reach-test-modified-functional-reach-test

Graf, C. G. (2008, April). Lawton—Brody Instrumental Activities of Daily Living Scale (I.A.D.L.). *Alz.Org*. Retrieved September 5, 2021, from https://www.alz.org/careplanning/downloads/lawton-iadl.pdf

Halabchi, F., Alizadeh, Z., Sahraian, M. A., & Abolhasani, M. (2017). Exercise prescription for patients with multiple sclerosis; potential benefits and practical recommendations. *BMC Neurology, 17*(1). https://doi.org/10.1186/s12883-017-0960-9

Hobbs, M. The role of occupational therapy in pulmonary rehabilitation, continuing education for occupational therapists. *Pdhacademy.Com*. PDH Academy. https://pdhacademy.com/wp-content/uploads/2016/11/PROOF3_117164_PDHAcademy_OT_ROLE-OF-OT-IN-PULMONARY-REHAB.pdf. Accessed February 6, 2021.

Jain, S. (2021, June 20). Glasgow Coma Scale—StatPearls—NCBI Bookshelf. *NCBI*. Retrieved September 5, 2021, from https://www.ncbi.nlm.nih.gov/books/NBK513298/

Katz Index of Independence in Activities of Daily Living. (2016, December 1). *Shirley Ryan AbilityLab*. Retrieved September 5, 2021, from https://www.sralab.org/rehabilitation-measures/katz-index-independence-activities-daily-living

Kohlman Evaluation of Living Skills. (2019, April 26). *Shirley Ryan AbilityLab*. Retrieved September 5, 2021, from https://www.sralab.org/rehabilitation-measures/kohlman-evaluation-living-skills

Lewis, S. M., Dirksen, R. R. S. N., Heitkemper, M. M. L., Bucher, L., Harding, M. M., Kwong, J., & Roberts, D. (2017). *Medical-Surgical Nursing*. Elsevier Gezondheidszorg.

Lin, K. (2020, August 30). Ranchos Los Amigos—StatPearls—NCBI Bookshelf. *NCBI*. Retrieved September 5, 2021, from https://www.ncbi.nlm.nih.gov/books/NBK448151/

Lopez, O. L., & Kuller, L. H. (2019). Epidemiology of aging and associated cognitive disorders: Prevalence and incidence of

Alzheimer's disease and other dementias. *Handbook of Clinical Neurology*, 139–148. https://doi.org/10.1016/b978-0-12-804766-8.00009-1

McCraith, D. (2016). ACLS-5 and LACLS-5 Test: Psychometric Properties and Use of Scores for Evidence-Based Practice. Allen Cognitive Group. allencognitive.com.

MoCA—Cognitive Assessment. (n.d.). *MoCA—Cognitive Assessment*. Retrieved September 5, 2021, from https://www.mocatest.org/

Moreno-Torres, I., Sabín-Muñoz, J., & García-Merino, A. (2019). CHAPTER 1. Multiple sclerosis: Epidemiology, genetics, symptoms, and unmet needs. *Drug Discovery*, 1–32. https://doi.org/10.1039/9781788016070-00001

Morgan, B. (n.d.). *Spinal Cord Functioning at C3 | LHSC*. London Health Sciences Centre. Retrieved November 8, 2021, from https://www.lhsc.on.ca/critical-care-trauma-centre/spinal-cord-functioning-at-c3

Muntges, L. (n.d.). *Acute care back to the basics: Vision assessment and management*. occupational therapy.com.

Occupational therapy practice framework: Domain and process—Fourth Edition. (2020, August 1). *American Journal of Occupational Therapy*. Retrieved September 5, 2021, from https://ajot.aota.org/article.aspx?articleid=2766507

O'Sullivan, S. B., Schmitz, T. J., & Fulk, G. D. (2019). *Physical Rehabilitation*. F.A. Davis Company.

Oxford Medical Education. (2016, April 15). *Mini-mental state examination (MMSE)*. Oxford Medical Education. Retrieved September 5, 2021, from https://oxfordmedicaleducation.com/geriatrics/mini-mental-state-examination-mmse/

Palmer, M. L., & Epler, M. E. (1998). *Fundamentals of Musculoskeletal Assessment Techniques* (2nd ed.). LWW.

Pendleton, H., & Schultz-Krohn, W. (2017). *Pedretti's occupational therapy: Practice skills for physical dysfunction (Occupational Therapy Skills for Physical Dysfunction (Pedretti))* (8th ed.). Mosby.

Performance Assessment of Self-Care Skills. (2015, June 5). *Shirley Ryan AbilityLab*. Retrieved September 5, 2021, from https://www.sralab.org/rehabilitation-measures/performance-assessment-self-care-skills

Reliability and validity of the mCTSIB dynamic platform test to assess balance in a population of older women living in the community. (2020). *PubMed Central (PMC)*. Retrieved September 5, 2021, from https://www.ncbi.nlm.nih.gov/pmc/articles/PMC7288384/

Saint Louis University Mental Status Exam. (2019, May 15). *Shirley Ryan AbilityLab*. Retrieved September 5, 2021, from https://www.sralab.org/rehabilitation-measures/saint-louis-university-mental-status-exam

Shoemaker, M. J., Dias, K. J., Lefebvre, K. M., Heick, J. D., & Collins, S. M. (2020). Physical therapist clinical practice guideline for the management of individuals with heart failure. *Physical Therapy*, *100*(1), 14–43. https://doi.org/10.1093/ptj/pzz127

Stamm, T. A., Machold, K. P., Smolen, J. S., Fischer, S., Redlich, K., Graninger, W., Ebner, W., & Erlacher, L. (2002). Joint protection and home hand exercises improve hand function in patients with hand osteoarthritis: A randomized controlled trial. *Arthritis & Rheumatism, 47*(1), 44–49. https://doi.org/10.1002/art1.10246

The Homebound Requirement. Www.Medicareinteractive.Org. https://www.medicareinteractive.org/get-answers/medicare-covered-services/home-health-services/the-homebound-requirement. Accessed October 17, 2020.

Tinetti Test. (n.d.). *Physiopedia*. Retrieved September 5, 2021, from https://www.physio-pedia.com/Tinetti_Test

Towfighi, A., Ovbiagele, B., El Husseini, N., Hackett, M. L., Jorge, R. E., Kissela, B. M., Mitchell, P. H., Skolarus, L. E., Whooley, M. A., & Williams, L. S. (2016, December). Poststroke depression: A scientific statement for healthcare professionals from the American Heart Association/American Stroke Association. *AHA Journals*. Retrieved September 9, 2021, from https://www.ahajournals.org/doi/10.1161/STR.0000000000000113

Trombly, C. A., Radomski, M. V., & Latham, C. A. T. (2002). *Occupational Therapy for Physical Dysfunction*. Lippincott Williams & Wilkins.

Tzelepis, F., Sanson-Fisher, R., Zucca, A., & Fradgley, E. (2015). Measuring the quality of patient-centered care: Why patient-reported measures are critical to reliable assessment. *Patient Preference and Adherence*, 831. https://doi.org/10.2147/ppa.s81975

Udell, J. A., Zawi, R., Bhatt, D. L., Keshtkar-Jahromi, M., Gaughran, F., Phrommintikul, A., Ciszewski, A., Vakili, H., Hoffman, E. B., Farkouh, M. E., & Cannon, C. P. (2013). Association between influenza vaccination and cardiovascular outcomes in high-risk patients. *JAMA, 310*(16), 1711. https://doi.org/10.1001/jama.2013.279206

Weissberg, K. (2020, February). Dementia management: Techniques for staging and intervention [Slides]. *Occupationaltherapy.Com*. https://occupationaltherapy.com

INDEX

Page numbers followed by f indicate figures, followed by t indicate tables, and followed by b indicate boxes.